THE GLUCOSE REBELLION COOKBOOK

Tactics, Recipes, and Nutritional Uprisings to Overthrow Type 2 Diabetes

By: Dr. Khalid Saeed, D.O.

Legal Stuff (Because Apparently You Can't Just Torch the Food Pyramid Without a Lawyer Present)

Medical Disclaimer

This cookbook is for educational, informational, and highly opinionated purposes only. It is not a substitute for medical advice, diagnosis, or treatment. Yes, even if you like it more than your endocrinologist.

Before making any changes to your diet, medications, exercise plan, or glucose-monitoring strategy—especially if you're pregnant, nursing, taking medication, or managing a chronic illness—talk to your own doctor. The real one. The one with your medical chart and your lab results.

Reading this book does not make the author your physician. No copays, no paperwork, no awkward silence while taking blood pressure readings, no prostate exams. Just recipes, science, sarcasm, and the occasional motivational slap.

Translation—Your rebellion, your responsibility. If you challenge an experimental pancake stack to a duel and lose, that's on you.

Author's Disclosure

Dr. Khalid Saeed, D.O., is a board-certified physician and a diabetic rebel who got tired of garbage nutrition advice, glucose rollercoasters, and medical gaslighting. This book is built on a potent cocktail of clinical experience, personal rebellion, peer-reviewed science, and absolute disdain for "low-fat" muffins.

This book does not create, imply, or suggest a doctor-patient relationship. Unless you've been formally evaluated, signed HIPAA disclosures, and surrendered your insurance card while avoiding eye contact about your A1c, Dr. Saeed is not your physician. Educational snark ≠ medical responsibility.

The content in this book is not individualized medical advice. It is a blueprint, not a mandate. Take what works, question everything else, and don't email him because your cousin's friend's dog trainer had "the opposite result." Seriously.

Liability Disclaimer

The author and publisher disclaim all liability, loss, injury, metabolic mishaps, emotional spiral, or late-night tortilla binges that result from reading or applying this book. Your choices are your own. So are your carbs.

In other words—You're the captain of your metabolic pirate ship. If you run it into an iceberg made of mac-n-cheese, that's on you.

Copyright Notice
© 2025 Khalid Saeed, D.O.
ISBN: 979-8-218-75846-2
The Glucose Rebellion Cookbook™
All rights reserved.

No part of this book may be reproduced, stored, reposted, photocopied, recorded, excerpted, quoted out of context, or turned into a social media slideshow without prior written permission—except for brief quotations used in reviews, articles, academic discourse, or sarcastic memes with appropriate credit.

Copyright violators will be sentenced to a kale smoothie that tastes like lawn clippings while being lectured to by a cereal box mascot. You've been warned.

Trademarks, Satire, and Nominative Fair Use
This book contains parody, satire, commentary, and criticism—on food marketing, public health dogma, nutrition myths, diet culture, and any label that tries to sell you sugar disguised as "heart healthy."

All brand names, product terms, public health slogans, and food-related trademarks remain the property of their respective owners. Use of these names is nominative, educational, or satirical in nature and does not imply affiliation, endorsement, or sponsorship of any kind.

References to things like "the cereal aisle mafia," "sugar in a trench coat," or "glucose cosplay" are metaphors. If your brand feels personally attacked, consider whether it should be.

This book's content falls under fair use protections for commentary, education, and parody as provided by *U.S. copyright law (17 U.S.C. §107)* and reinforced by *Campbell v. Acuff-Rose Music, 510 U.S. 569 (1994)*. If you're still confused, ask a lawyer. Or a librarian. Or someone who remembers when snack bars had five ingredients instead of fifty.

Illustrations

All illustrations, diagrams, cover art, and satirical graphics are original works by the author, created for educational, humorous, and critical purposes. Any resemblance to specific products, packaging, fictional characters, or weaponized desserts is coincidental, transformative, and protected by parody law.

Humor Notice

If you're unsure whether this book is mocking your breakfast, your favorite snack brand, or your inner carb addict—the answer is probably "yes." And it's okay. Laughter is anti-inflammatory.

Credits

Author, Designer, and Illustrator: Khalid Saeed, D.O.

Scientific Citations & References: All referenced studies are from peer-reviewed journals, listed in full in the "References" section at the back of the book. Because yes—we brought receipts.

Special Thanks: To every patient, peer, reader, and rebel who ever said, "There has to be a better way." You were right. This is it.

ACKNOWLEDGMENTS

Every Rebellion Has Its Allies

No revolution happens in a vacuum. This book may be written with one voice, but it carries the echoes of many: mentors, colleagues, patients, friends, and a few gloriously stubborn beta-testers who refused to eat another bowl of "heart healthy" cereal.

To my patients—You showed up tired, foggy, inflamed, and discouraged—and then you rose. You said yes to science, to spice, to sanity. You became rebels in your own kitchens. Thank you for trusting me with your health, your stories, and your meal logs.

To my medical mentors—The ones who questioned conventional wisdom, cited real data, and weren't afraid to say, "Maybe we were wrong." You helped light the match that burned down the food pyramid.

To my friends and family—For tolerating my endless rants about insulin resistance, for pretending to like my cauliflower experiments, and for believing in this rebellion long before it had a title. You're the real MVPs of metabolic reform.

To the data—Every study, every chart, every n-of-1 that challenged the dogma and told the truth about food, insulin, and disease—you fueled every page of this book. Science, not slogans.

And finally—To every reader still in the trenches, still figuring it out, still daring to ask for more from their body and brain: keep going. You are the rebellion now. And this time, we're not giving it back.

DEDICATION

For every person who was told they were "non-compliant" instead of "under-informed."

For every patient who left the clinic with more questions than answers.

For everyone who' ever stared down a donut and said, "Not today, endocrine chaos."

This one's for the rebels.

The ones who asked "why," demanded "how," and refused to accept that chronic disease was their final draft.

May your forks be mighty, your blood sugar boring, and your spirit completely uncooperative with the status quo.

TABLE OF CONTENTS

Acknowledgments i
Dedication iii

Part I: The Glucose Rebellion Begins 7
Chapter 1: Burn the Food Pyramid 9
Chapter 2: Science Snapshot: Glucose and Insulin Explained 13
Chapter 3: The Glucose Rebellion Manifesto 17
Chapter 4: What Low Carb Actually Means (and Why Most People Get It Wrong) 23

Part II: Tactical Eating for Metabolic Victory 31
Chapter 5: How to Build a Rebel Meal 33
Chapter 6: Breakfasts That Don't Backfire 39
Chapter 7: Lunches That Keep You in the Game (Not in a Nap) ... 51
Chapter 8: Dinners That Don't End in Regret or Glucose Spikes ... 63
Chapter 9: Desserts That Don't Destroy Your Pancreas 75
Chapter 10: Snacks That Don't Ruin Everything 87
Chapter 11: Beverages That Don't Betray You 97
Chapter 12: Dips, Dressings, and Sauces That Won't Take You Down 103

Part III: Strategy, Survival, and Science 115
Chapter 13: Flavor Science for Rebels 117
Chapter 14: Grocery Store Guerrilla Tactics 123
Chapter 15: Kitchen Setup for the Blood Sugar Battle 129
Chapter 16: Exercise for People Who'd Rather Nap 135
Chapter 17: Rebel Psychology 141

Chapter 18: When the World Pushes Back..................................147
Chapter 19: The Long Game...153
Chapter 20: Final Rebel Thoughts..159

The Next Chapter (Pun Intended) 163
About the Author 165
References 167
Suggested Reading and Tools 177
Glossary for the Biochemically Bamboozled 181

PART I:
THE GLUCOSE REBELLION BEGINS

CHAPTER 1
BURN THE FOOD PYRAMID

Metabolic Lies, Glycemic Betrayal,
and the Science They Never Taught You

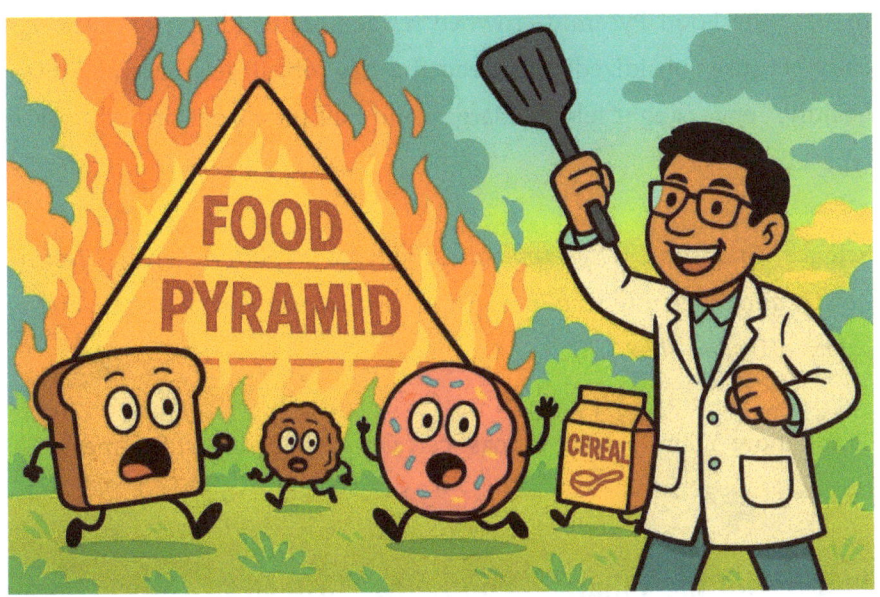

What You'll Learn

1. Why the original USDA Food Pyramid was less a nutrition guide and more a grain-marketing brochure.
2. How chronic carbohydrate overload drives insulin resistance long before fasting glucose tips into the "diabetic" range.
3. A tactical blueprint for torching legacy guidelines and replacing them with hormone-first eating rules.

Rebel Rallying Cry

If you "ate healthy" yet your continuous glucose monitor (CGM) graph looks like the EKG of a caffeinated hummingbird, you're not broken—you're **hoodwinked**. The system said six servings of bread kept hearts happy; instead, it kept insulin howling and pancreas overtime pay sky-high. Time to strike the match.

The Pyramid Scheme—Literally

In 1992 the Food Pyramid crowned refined grains king: 6–11 servings daily because subsidized corn needed a day job. Bagels became "heart healthy," eggs caught felony charges, and half the planet drifted toward type 2 diabetes.

Science Snapshot: *High-refined-carbohydrate patterns raise fasting insulin and accelerate insulin resistance within five years, independent of calories (Hall et al., 2018).*

Translation: Your "balanced" toast-cereal-banana breakfast is a metabolic prank.

You're Not the Villain—You're the Hostage

Follow the Pyramid for a week: spike, crash, snack, repeat. A decade later you're handed an Rx for Metformin. The system isn't broken; it's executing exactly what it was designed to do—move grain inventory, not safeguard hormones.

Science Snapshot: *Frequent post-prandial spikes raise triglycerides and visceral fat even in non-diabetics (Monnier & Colette, 2015).*

Translation: Snack aisles double as time-release fat storage.

Insulin Overdrive—When the Hall Monitor Never Clocks Out

Insulin is the firefighter; refined carbs are the arsonist. Keep alarms blaring and cells don noise-canceling headphones—hello, insulin resistance.

Science Snapshot: *Chronic hyperinsulinemia forecasts type 2 diabetes up to a decade in advance (Tabák et al., 2009).*

Translation: If insulin shouts all day, eventually nobody listens—and your pancreas buys a megaphone.

Metabolic Red-Flag Checklist

Red Flag	Why It Matters	Typical Pyramid Culprit
Post-lunch coma	Indicates reactive hypoglycemia	"Heart-healthy" sandwich + fruit juice
Mid-morning snack cravings	Insulin overshoot → glucose crash	Cereal + skim milk
Abdominal weight gain	Marker for compensatory hyperinsulinemia	Daily grain grazing
Triglycerides >150 mg/dL	Liver converting carbs → fat	"Low-fat" snack fest

"Improved" Guidelines—Same Lobbyists, New Icons

2005: Pyramid goes vertical, adds a stick figure sprinting up the side. 2011: MyPlate debuts, still starch-heavy, still missing a hormone column. Your glucometer is more honest than any federally funded infographic.

New Rule—Metabolic First, Macros Second

Ask of every bite: *What will this do to my hormones in the next two hours?* If the answer resembles insulin gymnastics, pass. Your mitochondria want a peaceful workday.

Exit Ramp—Strike the Match

The Food Pyramid isn't a meal plan; it's a tombstone for metabolic flexibility. Burn it, bury it, and grab a skillet.

Rebel Command (Chapter Recap)

1. Carbs aren't evil; chronic carb frequency is.
2. Insulin spikes are optional—industry profit isn't your biology's problem.
3. Any guideline that ignores hormones belongs in the trash heap with low-fat muffins.

CHAPTER 2
SCIENCE SNAPSHOT: GLUCOSE AND INSULIN EXPLAINED

The Hormonal Soap Opera That Happens Every Time You Eat Toast

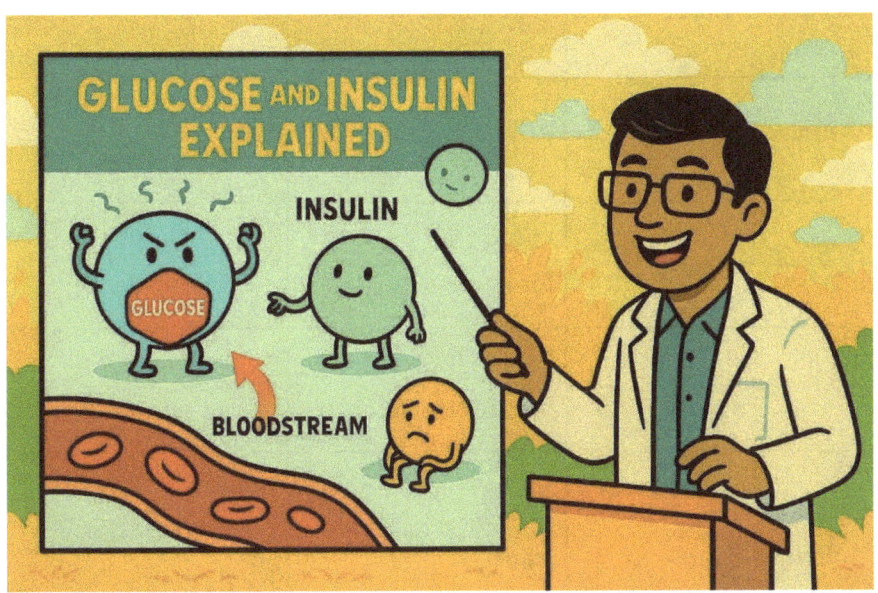

What You'll Learn

1. The minute-by-minute choreography of glucose, insulin, glucagon, cortisol, and friends.
2. Why identical granola bars can trigger wildly different spikes in two "healthy" people.
3. Tactical hacks—protein-first, mixed-macro, timing—that flatten the curve without spreadsheets.

Rebel Rallying Cry

Your bloodstream is a sleepy cul-de-sac until you toss in a croissant. Glucose floods the neighborhood, insulin sprints out like a bouncer, glucagon sulks in the corner. Understand the drama, and you can direct the script.

Meet the Cast

Role	Job Description	When It Becomes a Problem
Glucose	Primary cellular fuel	Chronic surplus = oxidative chaos
Insulin	Opens cellular doors for glucose	Too high, too often → cells go deaf
Glucagon	Signals liver to release stored fuel	Suppressed by perpetual snacking
Cortisol & Epinephrine	Emergency response team	Surge when glucose tanks after carb-only meals

Act I: The Granola Trap

- You eat a "healthy" granola bar:
- 20 min — Glucose spikes.
- 25 min — Insulin surges.
- 60 min — Glucose crashes.
- 90 min — Brain demands another snack.

Science Snapshot: *Post-spike crashes increase hunger, irritability, fatigue—even in non-diabetics (Benedict et al., 2011).*

Translation: Mood swings aren't a character flaw—they're biochemical boomerangs.

Metabolic Speed-Trap Chart

Food	Time to Spike	Glucose Impact
White bread	15 min	High and fast
Banana	25 min	Moderate-high
Lentils	50 min	Low and slow
Broccoli	N/A	Fiber with shoes

Insulin Resistance: When the Bouncer Gets Ignored

Chronic high insulin levels → receptor deafness → pancreas shouts louder → fat gain, fatigue, eventually type 2 diabetes.

Science Snapshot: *Insulin resistance precedes diabetes by 10–15 years and drives central adiposity (Shanik et al., 2008).*

Translation: Calories aren't the conversation—hormones are.

Protein & Fat: The Glucose Bodyguards

Add protein and fat, and that spike flattens like a pancake under a dumbbell.

Science Snapshot: *Mixed macro meals cut glycemic response 30–50 % versus carbs alone (Wolever et al., 1991).*

Translation: Eat protein first—it's biochemical crowd control.

Rebel Lab—DIY Glucose Experiment

1. Test breakfast A: oatmeal + banana.
2. Next day test breakfast B: three eggs + spinach + avocado.
3. Compare CGM or finger-stick curves.
4. Try not to swear at your former breakfast routine.

Blood Sugar Targets (for Humans, Not Robots)

Timing	Ideal	Red Flag
Fasting	70–90 mg/dL	>100 mg/dL
1 hr post-meal	<120 mg/dL	>140 mg/dL
2-3 hrs post-meal	Back to baseline	Still elevated

Exit Ramp

Glucose isn't evil. Insulin isn't your enemy. The modern snack-ified menu is. Now that you've decoded the cast, you're ready to write a new script.

Rebel Command

1. Spikes are optional; curves can be coached.
2. Protein-first, mixed-macro meals recruit glucagon, GLP-1, and satiety hormones to your side.
3. Data beats dogma—test, observe, adjust.

CHAPTER 3
THE GLUCOSE REBELLION MANIFESTO

Six Core Principles for Tactical, Blood-Sugar-Smashing Nutrition

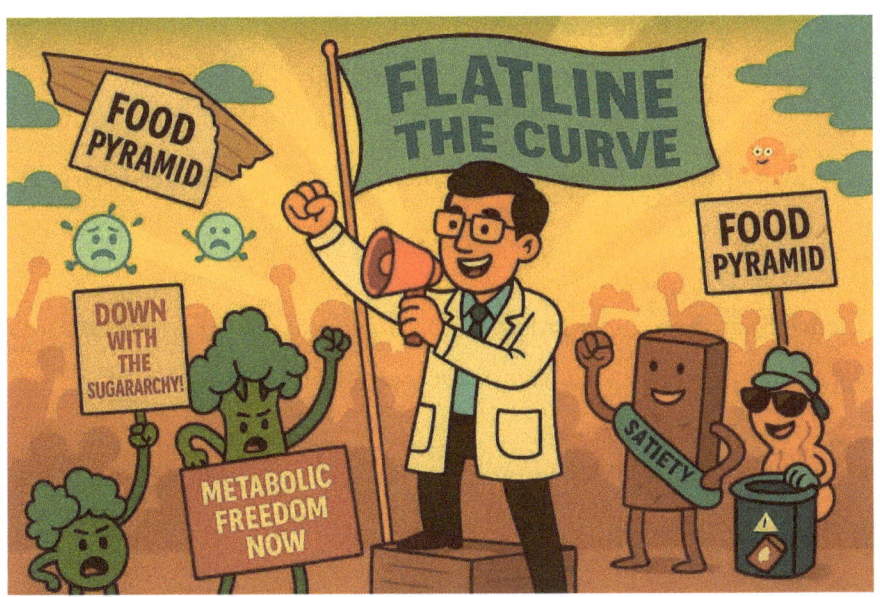

What You'll Learn

1. Why "eat better" is not a plan—structure beats motivation every time.
2. The six principles that restore hormonal sanity, crush cravings, and stabilize energy.
3. How to eat rebelliously without spreadsheets, starvation, or sad desk salads.

Rebel Rallying Cry

This isn't about dieting harder. This is about **opting out** of biochemical sabotage. Your body isn't broken—it's been hijacked by food systems optimized for shelf life, not metabolic life. These six principles are your tactical reboot protocol.

Program the Body, Don't Scold It

If your metabolism is behaving badly, check its instructions. You've been following advice from boxes with "heart healthy" stickers—designed by people more interested in quarterly reports than your pancreas.

Core Principle: Build meals from protein, fat, fiber, and micronutrients. Ditch barcodes.

Science Snapshot: *Ultra-processed foods drive excess calorie intake and glucose spikes—even when you're not hungry (Hall et al., 2019).*

Translation: If it looks like a science project, your mitochondria will panic accordingly.

Tame Insulin, Unleash Metabolism

Fat-burning doesn't happen when insulin's on patrol 24/7. You don't need to eliminate carbs entirely—unless your metabolism insists on it—but you do need to stop hand-feeding your glucose curve like a zoo animal.

Core Principle: Lower insulin-stimulating foods. Prioritize protein. Eat in defined windows.

Science Snapshot: *Low-carb diets reduce insulin, increase fat oxidation, and reverse type 2 diabetes (Hallberg et al., 2018; Unwin et al., 2016).*

Translation: Let insulin clock out so fat metabolism can clock in.

Use the Sun, Not a Snack Timer

Your circadian rhythm doesn't just control sleep—it sets your digestive efficiency. Night eating messes with your hormones like a 3 a.m. prank call.

Core Principle: Eat during daylight hours. Ditch the bedtime carb cuddle.

Science Snapshot: *Early time-restricted eating improves insulin sensitivity even without calorie reduction (Sutton et al., 2018).*

Translation: Late-night snacking is like asking your liver to process a cupcake with one eye closed.

Data > Dogma

Your glycemic response is not a group project. Generic advice assumes you're a textbook. You're not. You're a system with microbiota, stress, and sleep-debt variables.

Core Principle: Test. Observe. Adjust. Use a CGM, glucometer, or energy tracker.

Science Snapshot: *Glycemic responses to identical foods vary widely due to microbiome, stress, and circadian factors (Zeevi et al., 2015).*

Translation: Banana spike? That's personal—not universal.

Real Food Wins Every Audit

No health influencer ever outperformed a properly cooked egg. Real food speaks hormone. Fake food needs a label translator and a congressional lobbyist.

Core Principle: Eat food with roots, fins, faces, or a shelf life shorter than your last relationship.

Science Snapshot: *Whole food diets improve glucose control and lower inflammation—even without weight loss (Mozaffarian et al., 2020).*

Translation: If it needs an ad campaign, it probably needs a warning label too.

Structure Beats Motivation Every Time

Motivation is a mood. Structure is a system. You don't rise to the level of your willpower—you fall to the level of your prep.

Core Principle: Create defaults—prepped proteins, repeated meals, routine timing.

Science Snapshot: *Sustained behavior change requires structure and environment, not willpower (Wing & Phelan, 2005).*

Translation: Meal prep isn't cute—it's biochemical insurance.

Rebel Sidearm: Quick Reference Grid

Principle	Action	Biochemical Payoff
Protein-first	30g per meal minimum	Satiety, lower glucose
Carb-curated	≤15g net per meal	Lower insulin load
Time-gated eating	Finish by 7 p.m.	Better insulin sensitivity
Real food sourcing	Unprocessed only	Lower inflammation
Test, don't guess	CGM or glucometer	Personal precision
Default prep	Weekly protein batch	Fewer impulse carbs

Exit Ramp

This isn't about keto cosplay or orthorexic rules. This is about metabolic leverage. These six principles are how you get off the blood sugar rollercoaster—not by dieting harder, but by eating smarter.

Rebel Command

1. Your body isn't misbehaving. It's obeying a system designed for snacks.
2. Real change requires systems, not slogans.
3. Every meal is a metabolic message. Choose wisely, not perfectly.

CHAPTER 4
WHAT LOW CARB ACTUALLY MEANS (AND WHY MOST PEOPLE GET IT WRONG)

Spoiler: It's Not About Eating Butter Like a Barbarian

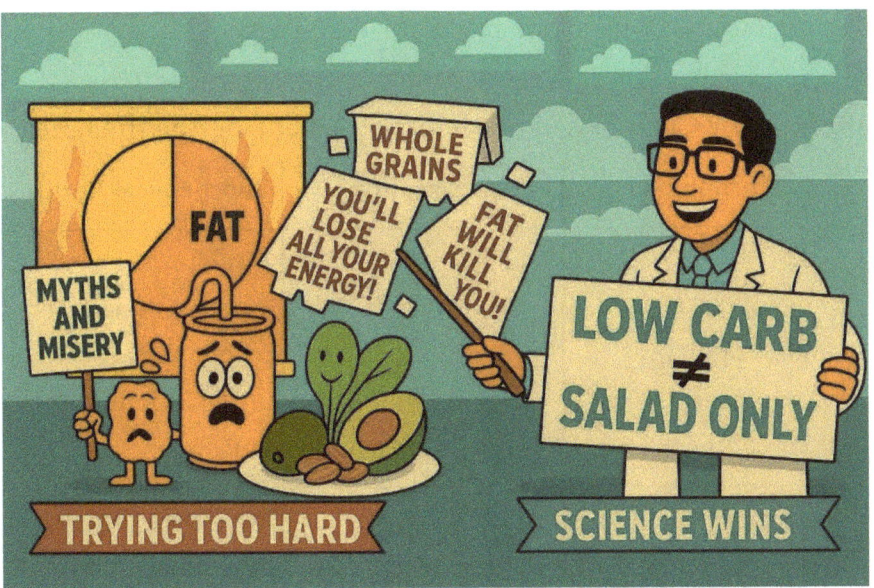

What You'll Learn

1. The actual definition of "low carb" and why most social media versions are junk.
2. The science behind why carbohydrate reduction works—not just for diabetes, but for energy, hunger, and hormones.
3. How to avoid common low-carb fails—like turning every snack into a cheese covered loophole of denial.

Rebel Rallying Cry

Low carb isn't a cult, a dare, or a personality. It's a strategy. It's about taming insulin—the drama queen hormone that's been hijacking your metabolism since the Food Pyramid told you six servings of bread was "heart-healthy." Somewhere along the way, it got hijacked by steak-only bros, keto cheesecake influencers, and oat milk evangelists.

The Carb Lanes (Pick Your Battlefield)

Here's the truth: carbs aren't inherently evil. They're just sneaky double agents. What matters isn't whether you *like* them—It's what they do to your hormones. Think of carb intake as lanes on a metabolic highway.

What "Low Carb" Really Refers To — Let's define the lanes:

Carb Intake	Description	Biochemical Reality
250–350g/day	Standard American Diet (SAD)	Insulin never clocks out. Fat storage gets tenure. Energy is unstable, hunger is loud.
100–150g/day	Moderate carb ("still-sorta-sugary")	You'll feel virtuous… right up until your CGM tattles on your sandwich.
50–100g/day	Low carb	Where hunger calms, glucose flattens, and insulin finally takes a coffee break.

What Low Carb Actually Means

Carb Intake	Description	Biochemical Reality
<50g/day	Very low carb / Ketogenic	Metabolic rehab mode. Fat burning reboots. Your pancreas sends you thank-you notes.
<30g/day	Insulin Zen Zone	My personal sweet spot—strict enough to reverse Type 2 diabetes, livable enough that cauliflower rice didn't make me cry.

Rebel Tip: It's not about the number. It's about the outcome: lower insulin, flatter glucose, reduced hunger.

Science Snapshot: *Low-carb diets consistently improve glycemic control, lower insulin, and reduce body weight—even without calorie counting (Feinman et al., 2015).*

Translation: Unless you're a Tour de France cyclist, 300g of carbs a day is not fuel—it's sabotage.

Why Low Carb Works (No, It's Not Magic)

You cut carbs → glucose spikes flatten → insulin drops → fat burning resumes → hunger normalizes → energy stabilizes.

Science Snapshot: *Reduced insulin leads to improved metabolic flexibility and appetite regulation (Hallberg et al., 2018).*

Translation: You're not eating less. You're finally eating sanely.

Where People Blow It (AKA Carb-Reduction Crimes)

Myth #1: Low Carb = No Carb

Vegetables are carbs. So are berries. The point is to eliminate *refined starches*, not act like spinach is contraband.

Common Fail: Fear of tomatoes. Meanwhile, oat milk lattes still happening.

Myth #2: Low Carb = Fat-Splattered Buffet

Just because you ditched bread doesn't mean crispy chicken skin smothered in mayonnaise is dinner.

Common Fail: Forgetting protein, fiber, and micronutrients. Deep-fried denial isn't a strategy.

Myth #3: "I Gave Up Bread but I Drink Smoothies"

Congratulations. You just liquefied the glycemic impact of a muffin.

Science Snapshot: *Smoothies and juice cause blood sugar spikes equal to soda (Basu et al., 2013).*

Translation: Liquid fruit is dessert in drag.

The Fiber Scam: Net Carbs vs. Total Carbs

Marketers want you to believe:

Net Carbs = Total Carbs – Fiber – Sugar Alcohols

But that's not the whole truth.
- Not all fiber is metabolically inert (inulin ≠ broccoli)
- Sugar alcohols often spike insulin anyway
- Some brands just lie

Rebel Tip: If a "3g net carb" bar has 27g of total carbs and tastes like cake—it's a scam with a fiber toupee.

Cosmetic Carb Cutting: The Halfway Failures

"Healthy" Move	Reality
No bun, but still eat fries	Still spiking
Skip toast, drink oat milk	Glucose ambush in a mug
Swap white rice for quinoa	Slightly slower spike—but still a spike
Paleo granola with honey	Granola + branding = breakfast candy

Science Snapshot: *Granola and health bars often spike glucose as much as conventional sweets (Bell et al., 2015).*

Translation: If the packaging is rustic, the sugar still counts.

What You Eat Instead (Yes, It's Still Delicious)

Food Group	Why It Works
Protein (eggs, tofu, meat)	Builds muscle, regulates appetite
Healthy fats (avocado, olive oil, nuts)	Satiety, hormone support
Low-carb veg (spinach, broccoli)	Fiber, micronutrients, glucose control
Optional carbs (berries, legumes)	If tolerated and dosed with care

Science Snapshot: *High-protein, low-refined-carb diets improve insulin sensitivity and inflammatory markers (Mozaffarian et al., 2018).*

Translation: Steak + greens = control. Granola + guilt = relapse.

Metabolic Results > Food Labels

Don't obsess over hitting 47.5g of carbs instead of 50. Ask:

- Am I hungry two hours after eating?
- Is my energy stable or flatlining?
- Does my CGM graph look like an EKG on roller skates?

Rebel Tip: If a food needs to tell you it's low carb, it probably isn't.

Exit Ramp

Low carb is not about punishment. It's about ending the hostage crisis in your bloodstream. You don't need dogma. You need data, hormone sanity, and meals that leave you unfazed instead of unconscious.

Rebel Command

1. Low carb isn't about extremes. It's about stability.
2. Fiber isn't a free pass. Labels lie—your CGM doesn't.
3. Swap the carb costume party for actual clarity.

PART II:
TACTICAL EATING FOR METABOLIC VICTORY

CHAPTER 5
HOW TO BUILD A REBEL MEAL

Why Your Food Should Have Delts and a Backstory

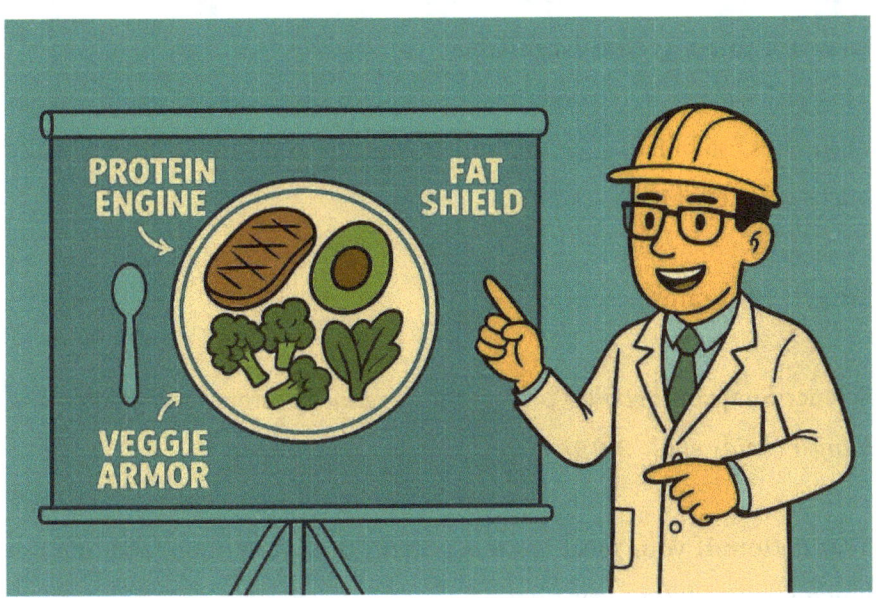

What You'll Learn

1. How to build a complete, low-carb plate that fuels instead of flattens you.
2. Why protein is non-negotiable, carbs are guests not hosts, and fat is your strategic ally.
3. How to turn your kitchen into a metabolic command center—not a snack disaster zone.

Rebel Rallying Cry

This isn't about sad salads or boiled chicken. You're not here for diet misery cosplay. You're here to weaponize your plate. Done right, your meal doesn't just fill you up—it flattens cravings, sharpens thinking, and tells insulin to take the afternoon off.

The Three Laws of a Rebel Meal

Law #1: Protein Is Non-Negotiable

This isn't a garnish. It's your anchor. Protein slams the brakes on hunger hormones, stabilizes glucose, and builds the only tissue that actually burns calories at rest—muscle.

Target: 30+ grams per meal

Science Snapshot: *Higher-protein meals reduce postprandial glucose and hunger (Leidy et al., 2015).*

Translation: If your meal has less protein than your cat's food, it's not lunch—it's a blood sugar prank.

Law #2: Carbs Must Apply for a Visa

Carbs aren't banned. They're vetted. No entry without fiber, nutrients, and proof they won't hijack your pancreas.

Approved examples: lentils, berries, leafy greens

Denied at the border: cereal, oat milk, dried fruit disguised as "natural"

Law #3: Fat Is Your Ally, Not a Villain

Fat doesn't make you fat. It makes you full, happy, and hormonally intact.

Science Snapshot: *Dietary fat, when paired with protein and fiber, flattens glycemic response (Wolever et al., 1991).*

Translation: Olive oil is not the enemy. Fat-free crackers are.

The Rebel Plate Blueprint

Plate Section	Function	Example Foods
½ Plate: Protein + Non-Starchy Veg	Satiety, micronutrients, muscle fuel	Eggs, chicken, tofu + spinach, peppers
¼ Plate: Healthy Fats	Hormonal support, flavor	Olive oil, nuts, avocado, full-fat dairy
¼ Plate (Optional): Slow Carbs	Fiber and minimal glucose chaos	Lentils, berries, roasted squash

Why Protein Comes First (Always)

Start with protein, and everything else behaves. It triggers GLP-1 (Glucagon-Like Peptide-1) and PYY (Peptide YY) hormones—your hunger bouncers—and it minimizes insulin's dramatic entrance.

Goal: 1.2–2.0 g protein/kg body weight/day

Meal Minimum: 30g protein per sitting

Science Snapshot: *Protein-first sequencing reduces glucose spikes in mixed meals (Jakubowicz et al., 2013).*

Translation: Eat the steak. Then decide if you even need the berries.

The Buildable Template

- **Start with Protein:** eggs, salmon, tempeh, tofu, sardines, turkey
- **Add Non-Starchy Veg:** greens, peppers, cauliflower, mushrooms
- **Layer Healthy Fats:** olive oil, tahini, avocado, nuts
- **Optional Carb Component:** ≤15g net carbs from berries, lentils, etc. (if tolerated)

Fiber: The Unsung Hero

Forget label-fiber and bar-fiber. You want plant-embedded, metabolically active fiber.

Top sources: cruciferous veg, leafy greens, chia, psyllium

Science Snapshot: *Natural dietary fiber improves insulin sensitivity and fasting glucose (Weickert & Pfeiffer, 2008).*

Translation: Fiber doesn't mean a nutrition bar. It means broccoli.

Rookie Mistakes to Avoid

Rookie Move	Reality Check
Skipping protein at breakfast	Coffee and carbs = glucose grenade
Mistaking lettuce for a meal	Where's the protein? Where's the fat?
Using fruit as the carb base	Berries = condiment, not main event
Fearing salt on low-carb	Sodium loss is real—season your food like you mean it

Real-World Showdown: The Disaster vs. The Rebel Plate

The Fail Plate

- Granola bar
- Low-fat yogurt
- Banana
- *Macros:* Net Carbs: 90g | Protein: 12g | Fat: 2g
- *Outcome:* Spike → crash → snack → brain fog

The Rebel Plate

- 2 eggs cooked in olive oil
- 1 cup sautéed spinach
- A few blackberries
- Sprinkle of feta
- *Macros:* Net Carbs: 8g | Protein: 30g | Fat: 22g
- *Outcome:* No crash, no cravings, no regret

Science Snapshot: *High-protein, fat-inclusive breakfasts flatten insulin and increase energy (Jakubowicz et al., 2013).*

Translation: Start your day with actual fuel, not marketing fiction.

Meal Frequency: Fewer, Stronger Meals Win

Structure	Benefits
2–3 meals per day	Lower insulin exposure, more satiety
No snacks unless necessary	Prevents grazing-induced spikes
Focused meal windows	Supports circadian alignment

Rebel Tip: You're not a squirrel. Stop foraging every two hours.

Exit Ramp

A rebel meal is simple: protein, fiber, fat. If your plate doesn't do those three things, it's not helping you—it's helping Big Snack. Start strong, finish smarter.

Rebel Command

1. Meals should support muscle, not munchies.
2. Protein is a strategy, not a side dish.
3. Your plate isn't just food—it's a hormone intervention.

4.

CHAPTER 6
BREAKFASTS THAT DON'T BACKFIRE

Metabolically Tactical Ways to Start the Day

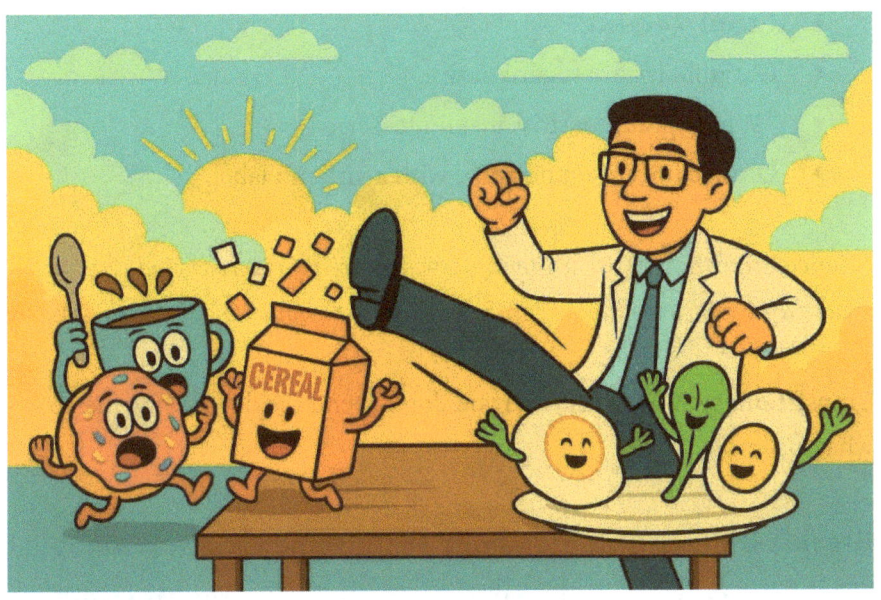

What You'll Learn

1. Why most "healthy" breakfasts are just glucose grenades with good PR.
2. How to build a breakfast that stabilizes energy, ends cravings, and keeps insulin quiet.
3. 15 fully-armed, low-carb breakfast recipes that fuel your rebellion.

Rebel Rallying Cry

If you start your day with sugar, don't act surprised when you're exhausted by 10 a.m. raiding the vending machine like a raccoon in a food court. Your metabolism deserves better. Breakfast should launch your day, not sabotage it.

The Morning Metabolic Crime Scene

- Cereal = dessert.
- Oat milk latte = sugar bomb.
- "Whole grain toast" = insulin teaser.
- Orange juice = liquid spike with a vitamin label.

Science Snapshot: *High-protein, low-carb breakfasts reduce daily caloric intake and improve glucose control for up to 24 hours (Leidy et al., 2007).*

Translation: Win breakfast, and you don't spend the day playing metabolic whack-a-mole.

Breakfast Blueprint: Metabolic Requirements

Metric	Minimum Target	Why It Matters
Protein	30g	Shuts down ghrelin, fuels muscle
Net Carbs	≤15g	Prevents glucose rollercoasters
Fat	≥15g	Slows digestion, stabilizes energy
Fiber	Real food sources only	Supports satiety, glucose control

Rebel Breakfast #1 — Three-Egg Spinach Power Bowl
Ingredients
- 3 eggs
- 1 cup spinach
- 1 tbsp olive oil
- Salt, pepper, chili flakes

Instructions: Scramble eggs in olive oil. Add spinach halfway through. Season with rebellion.

Macros: Net Carbs: 6g | Protein: 28g | Fat: 26g

Science Snapshot: *Leafy greens reduce fasting insulin (Blekkenhorst et al., 2018).*

Translation: Your body wants spinach, not cereal mascots.

Rebel Breakfast #2 — Turkey-Avocado Wake-Up Wrap
Ingredients
- 2 oz nitrate-free turkey
- ½ avocado
- 1 low-carb tortilla
- Spinach, mustard, herbs

Instructions: Assemble, roll, devour like you're on a mission.

Macros: Net Carbs: 9g | Protein: 30g | Fat: 22g

Science Snapshot: *Avocados improve insulin sensitivity (Wang et al., 2015).*

Translation: Guac isn't extra if it prevents diabetes.

Rebel Breakfast #3 — Cottage-Chia Crunch Bowl

Ingredients

- ½ cup full-fat cottage cheese
- 1 tbsp chia seeds
- 1 tbsp walnuts
- A few berries (optional)

Instructions: Stir. Chill for 10 minutes. Eat slowly. Feel smug.

Macros: Net Carbs: 8g | Protein: 24g | Fat: 18g

Science Snapshot: *Chia reduces post-meal glucose (Vuksan et al., 2010).*

Translation: Tiny seeds, big glucose payoff.

Rebel Breakfast #4 — Green Eggs (with Kale)

Ingredients

- 2 eggs
- ¼ cup chopped kale
- 1 tbsp ghee
- Garlic powder

Instructions: Sauté kale in ghee. Scramble in eggs. Serve sarcastically.

Macros: Net Carbs: 5g | Protein: 18g | Fat: 17g

Science Snapshot: *Leafy greens lower BP and fasting glucose (Blekkenhorst et al., 2018).*

Translation: Eat your greens. Fight your spikes.

Rebel Breakfast #5 — Flaxseed Waffles That Lift

Ingredients

- 1 egg
- 1 tbsp ground flaxseed
- 1 tbsp almond flour
- Dash vanilla
- Water to thin

Instructions: Mix. Pour into waffle iron. Skip syrup, keep pride.

Macros (2 waffles): Net Carbs: 4g | Protein: 11g | Fat: 14g

Science Snapshot: *Flax reduces fasting glucose in type 2 diabetes (Pan et al., 2007).*

Translation: Waffles can work—if they aren't made of sugar and shame.

Rebel Breakfast #6 — Protein-First Berry Shake

Ingredients

- 1 scoop whey or plant protein
- ½ cup almond milk
- ¼ cup frozen berries
- 1 tbsp flaxseed
- Ice

Instructions: Blend until smooth. Serve when your pancreas needs backup.

Macros: Net Carbs: 7g | Protein: 30g | Fat: 15g

Science Snapshot: *Protein shake breakfasts lower glucose and insulin (Wang et al., 2008).*

Translation: Shakes are fine—if they're not milkshakes in disguise.

Rebel Breakfast #7 — Smoked Salmon & Avocado Stack

Ingredients

- 2 oz smoked salmon
- ½ avocado
- 1 boiled egg
- Capers, lemon, black pepper

Instructions: Stack and devour like a bagel's smarter cousin.

Macros: Net Carbs: 3g | Protein: 18g | Fat: 21g

Science Snapshot: *Omega-3s reduce fasting insulin and inflammation (Balk et al., 2006).*

Translation: Fatty fish = metabolic win.

Rebel Breakfast #8 — Carb-Controlled Huevos Rancheros

Ingredients:

- 2 eggs
- ¼ cup sugar-free salsa
- ¼ avocado
- 1 low-carb tortilla (if tolerated)

Instructions: Cook eggs. Top with salsa, avocado. Serve on tortilla (or lettuce wrap).

Macros: Net Carbs: 11g | Protein: 27g | Fat: 19g

Science Snapshot: *Fat and fiber slow glucose absorption (Wolever et al., 1991).*

Translation: Breakfast doesn't need to spike your CGM to taste like a celebration.

Rebel Breakfast #9 — Greek Omelet Muffins (makes 4)

Ingredients:

- 4 eggs
- ¼ cup crumbled feta
- Chopped spinach, olives
- Oregano

Instructions: Whisk, pour into muffin tin. Bake at 350°F for 18–20 minutes.

Macros (per muffin): Net Carbs: 2g | Protein: 8g | Fat: 6

Science Snapshot: *Protein at breakfast lowers calorie intake the rest of the day (Leidy et al., 2007).*

Translation: Portable eggs prevent pastry regret.

Rebel Breakfast #10 — Savory "Noats" Porridge

Ingredients:
- 2 tbsp hemp hearts
- 1 tbsp chia
- 1 tbsp almond flour
- Water or almond milk
- Salt, herbs, turmeric

Instructions: Mix, heat, eat like the rebel you are.

Macros: Net Carbs: 8g | Protein: 21g | Fat: 23g

Science Snapshot: *Low-carb porridge improves satiety and flattens glucose (Noakes et al., 2014).*

Translation: Comfort food doesn't have to wreck your hormones.

Rebel Breakfast #11 — Tofu-Veggie Stir-Fry

Ingredients:

- ½ block firm tofu
- Zucchini, mushrooms, peppers
- 1 tbsp coconut aminos
- Sesame oil

Instructions: Sauté. Season. Serve hot.

Macros: Net Carbs: 7g | Protein: 17g | Fat: 14g

Science Snapshot: *Plant protein supports glucose control and lean mass (Fukagawa et al., 1990).*

Translation: Plants can hit macros too.

Rebel Breakfast #12 — Sardine & Olive Tapenade Plate

Ingredients:

- 1 tin sardines in olive oil
- 5–6 olives
- Cucumber slices
- 1 boiled egg

Instructions: Arrange like a breakfast charcuterie board. Own it.

Macros: Net Carbs: 4g | Protein: 23g | Fat: 17g

Science Snapshot: *Sardines improve fasting glucose and triglycerides (Di Giuseppe et al., 2014).*

Translation: Smells weird. Works beautifully.

Rebel Breakfast #13 — Peanut-Cacao Chia Parfait
Ingredients:
- 2 tbsp chia seeds
- ½ cup almond milk
- 1 tbsp natural peanut butter
- 1 tsp cacao nibs

Instructions: Soak chia overnight. Top with natural peanut butter and cacao.

Macros: Net Carbs: 10g | Protein: 12g | Fat: 21g

Science Snapshot: *Cacao flavonoids improve insulin sensitivity (Shrime et al., 2011).*

Translation: You get chocolate. Your pancreas gets peace.

Rebel Breakfast #14 — Spicy Egg-Drop Soup Mug
Ingredients:
- 2 eggs
- 1 cup broth
- Chili oil, sesame, green onion
- Spinach

Instructions: Boil broth. Stir in eggs. Add greens. Sip like a rebel.

Macros: Net Carbs: 3g | Protein: 20g | Fat: 8g

Science Snapshot: *Protein-based soups suppress ghrelin (Douglas et al., 2014).*

Translation: Slurp away. You've earned this.

Rebel Breakfast #15 — Almond-Crust Mini Quiche (makes 6)

Ingredients:

- 3 eggs
- ¼ cup almond flour
- Spinach, mushrooms
- Olive oil

Instructions: Bake crust, fill with egg mix, bake again.

Macros (per mini): Net Carbs: 3g | Protein: 9g | Fat: 9g

Science Snapshot: *Nut-based crusts reduce insulin response (Luo et al., 2021).*

Translation: Still breakfast. Just not sad.

Quick-Access: Rebel Breakfast Audit

Breakfast Item	Verdict
Cereal (any kind)	Glucose ambush
Oat milk latte	Dessert in a cup
Banana alone	Spike bait
Protein + greens + fat	Tactical breakfast
Eggs + avocado	Victory with seasoning

Exit Ramp

If your breakfast leaves you hungry, sleepy, or already thinking about lunch—it failed. These meals don't just feed you. They **arm you** for the day ahead.

Rebel Command

1. Start the day with protein, not panic.
2. Sugar doesn't belong in your sunrise.
3. If it spikes you, ditch it. If it fuels you, repeat it.

CHAPTER 7
LUNCHES THAT KEEP YOU IN THE GAME (NOT IN A NAP)

Midday Meals That Won't Torpedo Your Afternoon

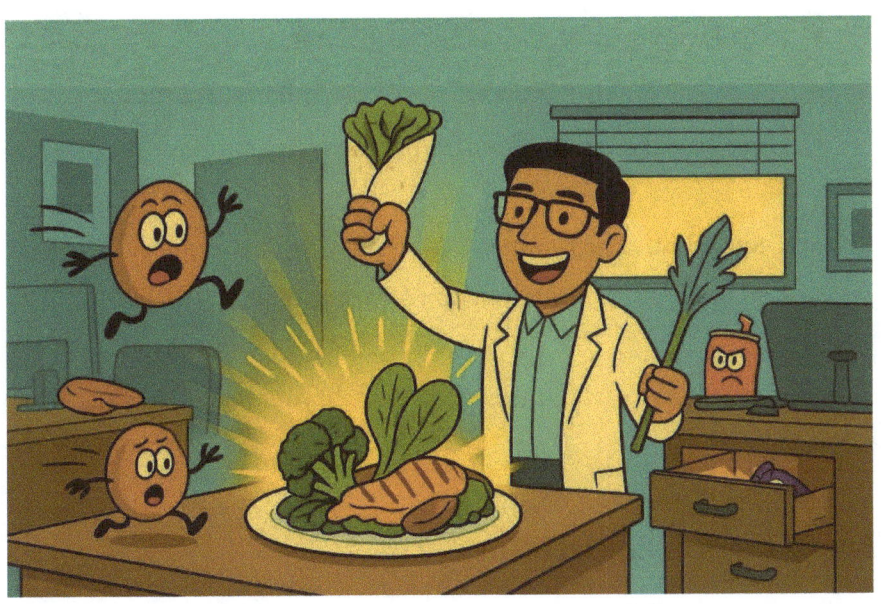

What You'll Learn

1. Why your lunch is often the hidden saboteur of your afternoon slump.
2. How to build a midday meal that delivers satiety, focus, and stable glucose.
3. 15 tactical, protein-forward lunches that actually work—no vending machine chasers required.

Rebel Rallying Cry

Lunch shouldn't leave you horizontal, brain-fogged, or on the internet searching for "healthy snacks" at 2:17 p.m. If your midday meal feels like a tranquilizer, it wasn't food—it was betrayal in a biodegradable box.

The Midday Metabolic Sabotage

Let's dissect the average lunch fail:

- Sandwich + fruit = carb sandwich
- Salad with no protein = sadness on a leaf
- "Low-fat yogurt + granola" = glucose spike with a spoon
- Fast-casual grain bowl = carb parade with branding

Science Snapshot: *High-protein, low-carb lunches reduce afternoon fatigue and improve cognitive function (Markus et al., 2010).*

Translation: If you're falling asleep after lunch, your insulin is whispering sabotage.

Lunch Rules of Engagement

Rule	Why
30g protein minimum	Shuts down afternoon hunger and brain drain
≤15g net carbs	No spike → no crash → no nap
Add fat on purpose	Satiety + flavor = compliance

Lunches That Keep You in the Game

Rule	Why
Fiber from plants	Not from wrappers labeled "heart healthy"
No grazing afterward	If your lunch needs a snack chaser, it failed

Rebel Lunch #1 — Chicken Caesar Lettuce Wraps

Ingredients

- 4 oz grilled chicken
- Romaine lettuce leaves
- Olive oil + lemon + mustard
- Parmesan, pepper

Instructions: Mix dressing. Layer ingredients. Wrap like a tactical taco.

Macros: Net Carbs: 5g | Protein: 32g | Fat: 22g

Science Snapshot: *Leafy greens improve insulin sensitivity (Blekkenhorst et al., 2018).*

Translation: You don't need croutons to call it lunch.

Rebel Lunch #2 — Spicy Tuna-Stuffed Avocados

Ingredients

- 1 can tuna (in olive oil)
- 1 ripe avocado
- Chili flakes, celery, salt

Instructions: Mix tuna. Fill avocado halves. Eat with spoon and swagger.

Macros: Net Carbs: 6g | Protein: 28g | Fat: 24g

Science Snapshot: *Avocados reduce inflammation and blunt post-meal glucose (Wang et al., 2015).*

Translation: Fat and fish—metabolic harmony.

Rebel Lunch #3 — Egg Salad Seaweed Rolls

Ingredients

- 2 boiled eggs
- 1 tbsp avocado oil mayo
- Nori sheets
- Cucumber sticks

Instructions: Make egg salad. Wrap in seaweed. Chill for crunch.

Macros: Net Carbs: 4g | Protein: 18g | Fat: 15

Science Snapshot: *Seaweed supports insulin sensitivity and gut health (Peng et al., 2015).*

Translation: This is sushi without sabotage.

Rebel Lunch #4 — Zoodle Pad Thai

Ingredients
- 1 zucchini, spiralized
- 3 oz chicken or shrimp
- 1 tbsp almond butter
- Coconut aminos, lime

Instructions: Cook protein. Stir-fry with zoodles and sauce.

Macros: Net Carbs: 10g | Protein: 26g | Fat: 20g

Science Snapshot: *Veggie noodle swaps reduce glycemic load (Brand-Miller et al., 2003).*

Translation: You can skip pasta and still win lunch.

Rebel Lunch #5 — Leftover Steak Salad

Ingredients
- 3 oz sliced steak
- Mixed greens
- Tomato, cucumber
- Olive oil + vinegar

Instructions: Assemble in bowl. Toss with defiance.

Macros: Net Carbs: 7g | Protein: 29g | Fat: 19g

Science Snapshot: *Red meat combined with dietary fiber significantly reduces postprandial glucose excursions (Johnston et al., 2002).*

Translation: Steak ≠ problem. Fries = problem.

Rebel Lunch #6 — Nori-Turkey Lunch Cones
Ingredients

- 3 oz turkey slices
- 1 nori sheet
- Avocado, cucumber
- Dash sesame oil

Instructions: Layer in nori. Roll like a cone. Eat like you're a stealth lunch ninja.

Macros: Net Carbs: 4g | Protein: 27g | Fat: 14g

Science Snapshot: *Lean protein paired with dietary fat enhances satiety while minimizing insulin response (Leidy et al., 2007).*

Translation: Wraps work better without wheat.

Rebel Lunch #7 — Greek Yogurt Chicken Slaw
Ingredients

- ½ cup shredded chicken
- ¼ cup plain Greek yogurt
- Cabbage slaw
- Garlic, lemon, dill

Instructions: Mix and chill. Eat like a tactical deli counter.

Macros: Net Carbs: 6g | Protein: 32g | Fat: 13g

Science Snapshot: *Yogurt lowers fasting glucose and supports gut flora (Marco et al., 2017).*

Translation: Chicken salad doesn't need sugar or mayo.

Rebel Lunch #8 — Egg Roll Bowl

Ingredients:

- 4 oz ground turkey or beef
- Shredded cabbage, carrots
- Coconut aminos, garlic, ginger

Instructions: Sauté meat. Add veg. Cook until softened. Stir to combine.

Macros: Net Carbs: 10g | Protein: 30g | Fat: 20g

Science Snapshot: *Cruciferous vegetables reduce inflammation and improve glucose uptake (Myzak et al., 2006).*

Translation: This tastes like takeout—but actually helps you stabilize your metabolism, not sabotage it.

Rebel Lunch #9 — Lentil-Lemon Protein Soup

Ingredients:

- ½ cup cooked lentils
- Chicken broth
- Lemon juice, parsley
- 1 scoop unflavored protein powder

Instructions: Heat broth and lentils. Stir in protein and seasonings.

Macros: Net Carbs: 13g | Protein: 28g | Fat: 8g

Science Snapshot: *Combining legumes and protein flattens glucose curves and supports satiety (Jenkins et al., 2012).*

Translation: Soup can actually work—if it's not 90% noodles.

Rebel Lunch #10 — Tofu Salad Power Plate

Ingredients:

- ½ block firm tofu
- Arugula, cherry tomatoes
- 1 tbsp tahini + lemon

Instructions: Slice tofu. Serve over greens with tahini drizzle.

Macros: Net Carbs: 7g | Protein: 22g | Fat: 17g

Science Snapshot: *Soy protein improves insulin response and preserves lean mass (Jayagopal et al., 2002).*

Translation: Meatless lunch doesn't mean low-protein lunch.

Rebel Lunch #11 — Tuna-Cucumber Stack

Ingredients:

- 1 can tuna
- ½ avocado
- Sliced cucumber
- Salt, paprika

Instructions: Mix tuna and avocado. Stack on cucumber slices.

Macros: Net Carbs: 5g | Protein: 30g | Fat: 21g

Science Snapshot: *Pairing lean protein with healthy fat reduces glycemic load (Wolever et al., 1991).*

Translation: Stack your protein. Ditch your bread.

Rebel Lunch #12 — Cauliflower Rice Burrito Bowl

Ingredients:

- ½ cup cauliflower rice
- 3 oz grilled chicken
- Guacamole, salsa
- Shredded lettuce

Instructions: Assemble like a burrito bowl. Eat with a fork and no regrets.

Macros: Net Carbs: 10g | Protein: 29g | Fat: 16g

THE GLUCOSE REBELLION COOKBOOK

Science Snapshot: *Non-starchy veggie swaps improve postprandial glucose (Brand-Miller et al., 2003).*

Translation: You can still have burritos—minus the blood sugar spike.

Rebel Lunch #13 — Eggplant Pizzas

Ingredients:

- Eggplant rounds
- Tomato paste
- Mozzarella
- Olive oil, basil

Instructions: Roast eggplant. Add toppings. Bake until bubbly.

Macros: Net Carbs: 9g | Protein: 17g | Fat: 14g

Science Snapshot: *Eggplant polyphenols reduce oxidative stress and improve glucose metabolism (Kwon et al., 2008).*

Translation: This is pizza that won't call your endocrinologist.

Rebel Lunch #14 — Shrimp and Zucchini Stir-Fry

Ingredients:

- 3 oz shrimp
- ½ zucchini, julienned
- Olive oil, garlic, lemon

Instructions: Sauté everything fast. Serve hot.

Macros: Net Carbs: 6g | Protein: 24g | Fat: 11g

Science Snapshot: *Shellfish has a lower insulin index than red meat (Uhe et al., 1992).*

Translation: Light protein doesn't mean light results.

Rebel Lunch #15 — Vegan Curry Chickpea Bowl

Ingredients:

- ¼ cup chickpeas
- ¼ cup full-fat coconut milk
- Cauliflower rice
- Curry powder, cumin, chili

Instructions: Simmer until thick and fragrant. Serve warm.

Macros: Net Carbs: 13g | Protein: 19g | Fat: 20g

Science Snapshot: *Legumes combined with fat and fiber blunt glucose spikes (Jenkins et al., 2012).*

Translation: Even chickpeas behave when you serve them with discipline.

Quick Audit: Lunch Landmines to Avoid

Food	Why It Fails
"Paleo" granola bowl	It's still a dessert.
Quinoa salad with raisins	Two carb types = double spike
Hummus + pita	Legume + starch = glucose party
Turkey sandwich on whole wheat	Bread still wins—blood sugar still loses
"Just a smoothie"	Translation: Liquid insulin spike

Exit Ramp

Lunch should not be a lullaby. These meals keep your head up, your glucose flat, and your insulin unbothered. You're not grazing. You're fueling with purpose.

Rebel Command

1. 30g protein. ≤15g net carbs. Repeat until confident.
2. If your lunch needs a snack, it's not lunch—it's a setup.
3. No grazing. No crashing. No compromises.

CHAPTER 8
DINNERS THAT DON'T END IN REGRET OR GLUCOSE SPIKES

Night Meals That Don't Wreck Your Hormones

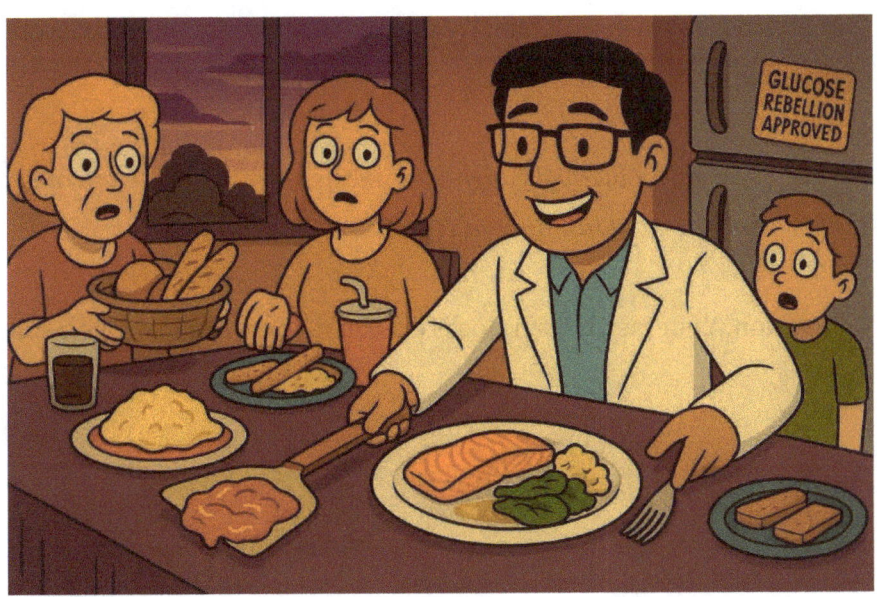

What You'll Learn

1. Why dinner is a metabolic ambush if you don't plan it right.
2. How to construct a nighttime meal that supports sleep, fat metabolism, and glucose control.
3. 15 tactical dinner recipes that don't spike your insulin or your shame.

Rebel Rallying Cry

Dinner shouldn't undo your day. But for most people, it does—glucose spikes, impulsive grazing, dessert disguised as dinner. The problem isn't your willpower. It's the system. This is where you flip the script and finish strong.

The Late Evening Glucose Ambush

You think you've been "good" all day, so you celebrate with pasta. But your metabolic system isn't built for 9 p.m. starch parties. Your pancreas has a bedtime. Respect it.

Science Snapshot: *Late-night high-carb meals impair glucose tolerance and increase overnight insulin levels (Morris et al., 2015).*

Translation: Your metabolism clocks out early—don't feed it like it's still working.

Dinner Rules of the Rebellion

Rule	Tactical Advantage
30g protein minimum	Muscle preservation, satiety, blood sugar stability
≤15g net carbs	Prevents glucose and insulin spikes before sleep
Fiber from actual plants	Slows digestion, feeds microbiome, flattens curve

Rule	Tactical Advantage
Fat on purpose	Supports hormonal balance and satisfaction
Zero grazing post-meal	Keeps overnight glucose in check and promotes fat oxidation

Rebel Dinner #1 — Lemon-Herb Roasted Chicken Thighs

Ingredients

- 2 bone-in chicken thighs
- Olive oil, lemon, thyme, garlic
- Side: roasted cauliflower

Instructions: Roast chicken at 400°F for 35–40 mins. Toss cauliflower in olive oil and roast alongside.

Macros: Net Carbs: 9g | Protein: 32g | Fat: 24g

Science Snapshot: *Dark meat paired with fiber-rich veg does not increase cardiovascular risk (Mozaffarian et al., 2010).*

Translation: Thighs are fine. So is flavor.

Rebel Dinner #2 — Seared Salmon with Broccoli and Tahini Drizzle

Ingredients

- 4 oz wild salmon
- 1 cup steamed broccoli
- 1 tbsp tahini, lemon, garlic

Instructions: Pan-sear salmon. Steam broccoli. Drizzle tahini sauce over both.

Macros: Net Carbs: 7g | Protein: 30g | Fat: 22g

Science Snapshot: *Omega-3s in salmon reduce insulin resistance (Balk et al., 2006).*

Translation: This is strategy, not indulgence.

Rebel Dinner #3 — Spaghetti Squash Bolognese
Ingredients
- 1 cup cooked spaghetti squash
- 4 oz ground turkey or beef
- Tomato paste, basil, garlic

Instructions: Brown meat. Stir in sauce. Serve over squash.

Macros: Net Carbs: 12g | Protein: 34g | Fat: 16g

Science Snapshot: *Vegetable swaps for pasta dramatically reduce glucose response (Brand-Miller et al., 2003).*

Translation: Comfort food, minus the carb coma.

Rebel Dinner #4 — Shrimp Stir-Fry with Bok Choy
Ingredients
- 3 oz shrimp
- Bok choy, red pepper
- Coconut aminos, ginger

Instructions: Sauté shrimp and veg in oil. Serve hot.

Macros: Net Carbs: 8g | Protein: 26g | Fat: 12g

Science Snapshot: *Shellfish has low insulin index, especially at night (Holt et al., 1997).*

Translation: Seafood = light protein, heavy on results.

Rebel Dinner #5 — Eggplant Lasagna Bake
Ingredients
- 1 eggplant, sliced
- ½ cup ground beef
- Tomato sauce, mozzarella, oregano

Instructions: Layer like lasagna. Bake at 375°F for 30 mins.

Macros: Net Carbs: 13g | Protein: 28g | Fat: 20g

Science Snapshot: *Low-carb lasagna variants significantly lower insulin and glucose (Gannon et al., 2004).*

Translation: You can still layer—just not with noodles.

Rebel Dinner #6 — Grilled Lamb Chops with Arugula Salad
Ingredients
- 2 small lamb chops
- Arugula, olive oil, lemon
- Shaved parmesan

Instructions: Grill lamb. Toss salad. Plate with zero apology.

Macro: Net Carbs: 6g | Protein: 33g | Fat: 25g

Science Snapshot: *Grass-fed lamb supports insulin sensitivity and provides CLA (Benjamin et al., 2000).*

Translation: It's not indulgent. It's smart meat.

Rebel Dinner #7 — Tofu Coconut Curry with Greens
Ingredients
- ½ block tofu
- Coconut milk, spinach, curry powder
- Garlic, turmeric

Instructions: Simmer tofu and greens in coconut curry. Serve warm.

Macros: Net Carbs: 10g | Protein: 21g | Fat: 22g

Science Snapshot: *Plant-based protein combined with dietary fat at dinner significantly reduces nocturnal glucose excursions (Kahleova et al., 2018).*

Translation: Curry can be cozy and tactical.

Rebel Dinner #8 — Zucchini Boats with Ground Chicken
Ingredients:
- 1 zucchini, halved and scooped
- 4 oz ground chicken
- Onion, tomato, spices

Instructions: Fill zucchini with cooked meat mixture. Bake at 375°F for 20 mins.

Macros: Net Carbs: 9g | Protein: 30g | Fat: 14g

Science Snapshot: *High-protein, low-carb veggie meals improve evening glucose tolerance (Cameron et al., 2009).*

Translation: Boats > bread bowls.

Rebel Dinner #9 — Stuffed Bell Peppers
Ingredients:
- 1 bell pepper, halved
- 3 oz ground beef or lentils
- Cauliflower rice, cumin, garlic

Instructions: Stuff and bake at 375°F for 25–30 mins.

Macros: Net Carbs: 11g | Protein: 27g | Fat: 15g

Science Snapshot: *Non-starchy stuffed meals stabilize glucose and improve satiety (Slavin, 2005).*

Translation: Dinner shouldn't come with a side of regret.

Rebel Dinner #10 — Tempeh Stir-Fry with Cashews
Ingredients:
- 3 oz tempeh
- Broccoli, red pepper
- 1 tbsp chopped cashews

Instructions: Sauté tempeh and veg. Add cashews at the end.

Macros: Net Carbs: 13g | Protein: 24g | Fat: 18g

Science Snapshot: *Fermented soy products improve glycemic control and reduce gut inflammation (Wang et al., 2016).*

Translation: This is what plant-based power looks like.

Rebel Dinner #11 — Cauliflower Gnocchi with Pesto Chicken

Ingredients:

- 1 cup cauliflower gnocchi
- 3 oz chicken breast
- Pesto (homemade or clean store-bought)

Instructions: Pan-sear gnocchi, add sliced chicken and pesto.

Macros: Net Carbs: 14g | Protein: 32g | Fat: 20g

Science Snapshot: *Low-glycemic dinner starches with protein stabilize evening glucose curves (Wolever et al., 2003).*

Translation: You can have a cozy meal without blood sugar sabotage.

Rebel Dinner #12 — Grilled Portobello Mushrooms with Mozzarella

Ingredients:

- 2 portobello caps
- Sliced mozzarella
- Basil, olive oil, balsamic drizzle

Instructions: Grill mushrooms. Top with cheese and herbs. Finish under broiler.

Macros: Net Carbs: 7g | Protein: 18g | Fat: 21g

Science Snapshot: *Mushrooms improve insulin resistance and antioxidant capacity (Valverde et al., 2015).*

Translation: You don't need meat to stabilize glucose—you need strategy.

Rebel Dinner #13 — Cabbage Steak with Spiced Ground Turkey

Ingredients:

- 1 thick cabbage slice
- 3 oz ground turkey
- Garlic, cumin, chili flakes

Instructions: Roast cabbage. Top with cooked turkey mixture.

Macros: Net Carbs: 8g | Protein: 28g | Fat: 16g

Science Snapshot: *Brassica vegetables enhance detox pathways and glucose utilization (Myzak et al., 2006).*

Translation: This isn't rabbit food—it's cellular warfare prep.

Rebel Dinner #14 — Sardine-Tomato Skillet with Kale

Ingredients:

- 1 tin sardines
- ½ cup diced tomatoes
- Kale, olive oil

Instructions: Sauté all together. Serve hot, with a side of confidence.

Macros: Net Carbs: 6g | Protein: 25g | Fat: 18g

Science Snapshot: *Sardines improve metabolic markers including glucose and lipid levels (Di Giuseppe et al., 2014).*

Translation: Strong smell, stronger results—because metabolic magic doesn't always smell like roses.

Rebel Dinner #15 — Baked Tofu with Brussels Sprouts and Mustard Glaze

Ingredients:

- ½ block tofu
- 1 cup Brussels sprouts
- Mustard, olive oil

Instructions: Roast tofu and sprouts at 400°F for 25 mins. Glaze with mustard mix.

Macros: Net Carbs: 10g | Protein: 24g | Fat: 20g

Science Snapshot: *Cruciferous veggies and plant protein improve insulin response and reduce visceral fat (Behzad et al., 2016).*

Translation: Bitter vegetables = sweet glucose results.

Metabolic Red Flags: The Dinner Edition

Problem	Cause
Night sweats	Late spike → insulin → hypoglycemia
Cravings before bed	Carb-heavy meal with no fat/protein
Waking up at 3 a.m.	Blood sugar crash after starchy dinner
Fatigue in morning	Insulin still elevated overnight

Exit Ramp

Dinner is where good intentions die—or get reinforced. You've made it this far. Don't let your evening meal reverse your entire day of stability. Eat to end the day flat (on your CGM, not your couch).

Rebel Command

1. Dinner should end your cravings, not start your spiral.
2. Protein + fiber + fat = hormonal bedtime story.
3. Save the indulgence fantasy. Your pancreas wants peace, not a pasta party.

CHAPTER 9
DESSERTS THAT DON'T DESTROY YOUR PANCREAS

Sweetness Without Sabotage

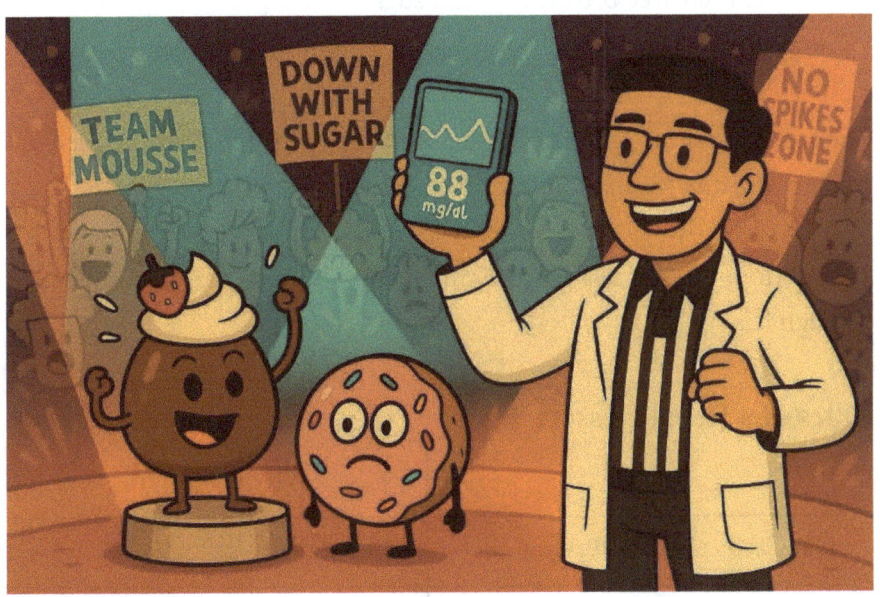

What You'll Learn

1. How to satisfy a sweet tooth without triggering a metabolic mutiny.
2. Which low-carb ingredients to embrace—and which "keto" traps to avoid.
3. 15 dessert recipes that deliver joy, not glucose trauma.

Rebel Rallying Cry

You don't have to swear off dessert like you joined a dietary monastery. But you do have to outsmart the sugar-industrial complex. Sweetness isn't evil. It's the way they've weaponized it that is.

The Dessert Delusion

Conventional desserts = nuclear glucose events.

- "All-natural" cookie = insulin trick
- "Gluten-free brownie" = still sugar
- "Keto bar" = check the label—it's often candy in drag

Science Snapshot: *Refined sugar and flour-based desserts increase triglycerides and insulin levels for hours (Ludwig, 2002).*

Translation: Dessert is a glucose minefield—but you can learn to dance through it.

Rules of a Rebel Dessert

Rule	Why It Matters
Net Carbs ≤7g per serving	Avoid glucose spikes
No hidden sugars	Look for erythritol, stevia, monk fruit—not maltitol
Must include fat or protein	Slows digestion, flattens spike
Real flavor or bust	Vanilla, cinnamon, cocoa, salt—don't skip the sensory experience
No sadness	If it tastes like punishment, you're doing it wrong

Rebel Dessert #1 — Chocolate Avocado Mousse

Ingredients

- 1 ripe avocado
- 2 tbsp cocoa powder
- 2 tbsp monk fruit sweetener
- Splash almond milk
- Pinch salt

Instructions: Blend until silky. Chill. Top with crushed nuts.

Macros: Net Carbs: 6g | Fat: 22g | Protein: 4g

Science Snapshot: *Avocado's monounsaturated fats slow carb absorption (Wang et al., 2015).*

Translation: It's creamy. It's smart. It's legal.

Rebel Dessert #2 — Almond Butter Coconut Balls

Ingredients

- ½ cup almond butter
- ¼ cup unsweetened shredded coconut
- 1 tbsp chia seeds
- 1 tbsp erythritol
- Dash vanilla

Instructions: Mix. Roll into balls. Refrigerate.

Macros (per 2): Net Carbs: 5g | Fat: 17g | Protein: 6g

Science Snapshot: *Almond butter and coconut provide healthy fats that support metabolic stability, while chia fiber helps blunt glucose spikes. Erythritol sweetens without impacting insulin (Munro et al., 1998).*

Translation: Fat-fueled dessert that flies under your pancreas's radar like a stealth snack.

Rebel Dessert #3 — Vanilla Chia Custard

Ingredients

- 1 cup unsweetened almond milk
- 2 tbsp chia seeds
- ½ tsp vanilla
- 1 tbsp stevia

Instructions: Mix. Chill overnight. Top with cinnamon.

Macros: Net Carbs: 4g | Fat: 8g | Protein: 6g

Science Snapshot: *Chia slows gastric emptying and reduces blood sugar rise (Vuksan et al., 2010).*

Translation: If pudding had morals, it would be this.

Rebel Dessert #4 — Peanut Butter Protein Fudge

Ingredients

- ½ cup natural peanut butter
- 2 scoops vanilla protein powder
- 1 tbsp coconut oil
- 2 tbsp erythritol

Instructions: Mix. Press into pan. Freeze until firm. Cut into squares.

Macros (per square):   Net Carbs: 3g | Fat: 14g | Protein: 10g

Science Snapshot: *Peanut butter brings healthy fats and a bit of fiber. Protein powder supports muscle maintenance and helps control hunger. Erythritol keeps it sweet without spiking blood sugar (Munro et al., 1998).*

Translation: The dessert that bench presses your cravings without benching your pancreas.

Rebel Dessert #5 — Lemon Cheesecake Bites

Ingredients

- ½ block cream cheese
- Zest + juice of ½ lemon
- 1 tbsp monk fruit sweetener
- 1 tbsp coconut flour

Instructions: Mix. Chill. Roll into bites.

Macros (2 bites)   Net Carbs: 6g | Fat: 16g | Protein: 5g

Science Snapshot: *Cream cheese delivers fat for satiety, while lemon adds flavor without sugar. Coconut flour provides a touch of fiber. Monk fruit sweetener keeps the glycemic impact near zero (U.S. FDA, 2010).*

Translation: Tart, rich, and unapologetically low-carb. Like cheesecake with a superiority complex.

Rebel Dessert #6 — Cinnamon Nut Mug Cake

Ingredients

- 1 egg
- 2 tbsp almond flour
- 1 tbsp crushed walnuts
- Dash cinnamon
- 1 tbsp monk fruit sweetener

Instructions: Mix in mug. Microwave 60–90 sec. Cool slightly.

Macros: Net Carbs: 5g | Fat: 14g | Protein: 9g

Science Snapshot: *Almond flour and walnuts offer healthy fats and fiber to slow glucose absorption. The egg adds protein for satiety. Monk fruit sweetener keeps it sweet without spiking insulin (U.S. FDA, 2010).*

Translation: Cake, if your pancreas wrote the recipe—low on sugar, high on self-respect.

Rebel Dessert #7 — Greek Yogurt Chocolate Bark

Ingredients
- ½ cup full-fat Greek yogurt
- 1 tbsp cocoa powder
- 1 tbsp chopped nuts
- Pinch salt
- Stevia to taste

Instructions: Spread on parchment. Freeze until solid. Snap into pieces.

Macros (per serving): Net Carbs: 6g | Fat: 9g | Protein: 10g

Science Snapshot: *Probiotics in yogurt may improve insulin sensitivity, while cocoa flavonoids support glucose metabolism. Fat and protein help blunt blood sugar spikes (Yadav et al., 2013; Grassi et al., 2005).*

Translation: Chocolate with probiotics—it tastes like dessert, but fights like medicine.

Rebel Dessert #8 — Berry-Almond Crisp

Ingredients
- ¼ cup mixed berries
- 1 tbsp almond flour
- 1 tbsp chopped almonds
- Cinnamon, butter, monk fruit

Instructions: Top berries with mixture. Bake 15 min at 375°F.

Macros: Net Carbs: 7g | Fat: 13g | Protein: 5g

Science Snapshot: *Berries are rich in polyphenols and fiber, which help reduce post-meal glucose spikes. Pairing them with fat and protein from almonds slows digestion and flattens the blood sugar curve (Törrönen et al., 2010).*

Translation: Dress your carbs in fat and fiber, and they behave. These berries showed up wearing an almond disguise—and your pancreas barely noticed.

Rebel Dessert #9 — Lemon Protein Pudding
Ingredients:
- 1 scoop unflavored protein
- ¼ cup coconut milk
- Lemon juice + zest
- Stevia

Instructions: Whisk protein powder with coconut milk. Add lemon juice, zest, and sweetener to taste. Chill 10–15 minutes.

Macros: Net Carbs: 4g | Protein: 20g | Fat: 10g

Science Snapshot: *Protein-based desserts improve postprandial glucose and preserve lean mass (Phillips et al., 2007).*

Translation: Dessert that doubles as recovery fuel.

Rebel Dessert #10 — Microwave Mug Cake (Almond Flour)

Ingredients:
- 2 tbsp almond flour
- 1 egg
- Cocoa, stevia, baking powder

Instructions: Mix in mug. Microwave 60–90 seconds.

Macros: Net Carbs: 8g | Protein: 9g | Fat: 14g

Science Snapshot: *Almond flour has minimal effect on blood sugar and adds fiber and magnesium (Chen et al., 2006).*

Translation: Dessert. One dish. No regret.

Rebel Dessert #11 — Zucchini Brownie Squares

Ingredients:
- ½ cup grated zucchini
- 1 egg
- Cocoa, almond flour, stevia

Instructions: Mix, bake at 350°F for 20 mins.

Macros (per square): Net Carbs: 9g | Protein: 5g | Fat: 10g

Science Snapshot: *Adding vegetables to baked goods lowers glycemic impact and adds fiber (Slavin, 2005).*

Translation: You just ate vegetables for dessert. Good job.

Rebel Dessert #12 — Ricotta Cocoa Swirl

Ingredients:
- ¼ cup whole-milk ricotta
- Cocoa powder
- Stevia, cinnamon

Instructions: Mix ricotta with cocoa, stevia, and a pinch of cinnamon until smooth. Chill or eat immediately with a smug grin.

Macros: Net Carbs: 5g | Protein: 7g | Fat: 10g

Science Snapshot: *Dairy protein and fat combo improves post-meal glucose and appetite regulation (Barr et al., 2000).*

Translation: Silky, sweet, and subversively blood-sugar friendly.

Rebel Dessert #13 — Frozen Protein Popsicles

Ingredients:
- 1 scoop vanilla protein
- Almond milk
- Berries (optional)

Instructions: Blend. Pour into molds. Freeze.

Macros: Net Carbs: 6g | Protein: 20g | Fat: 4g

Science Snapshot: *Cold, protein-rich snacks suppress appetite better than sugary frozen treats (Bellisle et al., 1997).*

Translation: You can have popsicles. You just can't be lazy about it.

Rebel Dessert #14 — Cinnamon "Sugar" Roasted Almonds

Ingredients:
- ¼ cup raw almonds
- Stevia, cinnamon
- Pinch salt, egg white

Instructions: Coat, bake at 325°F for 20 mins.

Macros: Net Carbs: 7g | Protein: 6g | Fat: 15g

Science Snapshot: *Almonds reduce post-meal glucose when consumed with or after carbohydrates (Josse et al., 2007).*

Translation: Dessert that multitasks like a pro.

Rebel Dessert #15 — Coconut-Lime Cream Cups

Ingredients:
- ¼ cup full-fat coconut milk
- Lime juice and zest
- Monk fruit

Instructions: Whisk and chill. Serve cold.

Macros: Net Carbs: 5g | Protein: 2g | Fat: 12g

Science Snapshot: *Medium-chain triglycerides in coconut aid fat metabolism and reduce glucose variability (St-Onge et al., 2003).*

Translation: Tropical. Tangy. Tactically sound.

Dessert Red Flags: Read the Label Like It's Lying (Because It Probably Is)

Phrase	Translation
"Keto-friendly"	Might have maltitol = spike town
"No sugar added"	May still contain fruit concentrates
"Natural"	Doesn't mean glucose-safe
"Low fat"	Translation: higher sugar
"Protein bar"	Check carbs - It might be a candy bar with abs

Exit Ramp

You're not a sugar monk. You're a rebel with standards. Dessert is allowed—but it answers to you now, not your cravings. Eat it on purpose, with science on your side.

Rebel Command

1. Sweetness is allowed. Sabotage is not.
2. Dessert must pass the protein-carb-fat audit.
3. No spikes. No shame. Just smarter indulgence.

CHAPTER 10
SNACKS THAT DON'T RUIN EVERYTHING

Emergency Fuel, Not a Lifestyle Choice

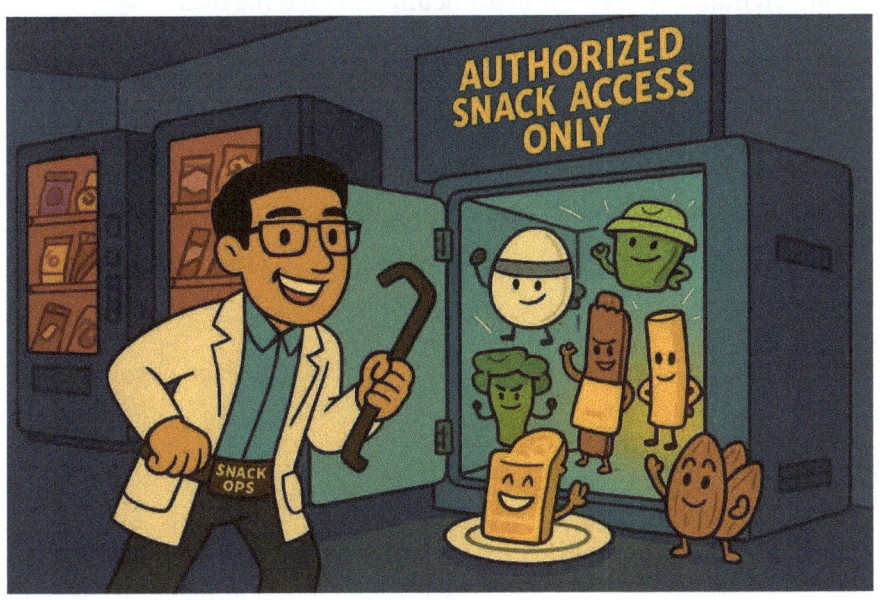

What You'll Learn

1. Why most snacking isn't hunger—it's hormonal chaos, boredom, or habit.
2. When to snack (rarely), how to snack (strategically), and what to snack on (not sadness in a plastic wrapper).
3. 15 low-carb, protein-forward snack options that won't detonate your glucose.

Rebel Rallying Cry

Snacking should be a contingency plan, not a constant state of eating. If you're "hungry" every two hours, you're not underfed—you're over-spiked. A properly built meal keeps you upright. A snack should be a tool, not a crutch.

The Snacking Delusion

What you think: "I need a little something to hold me over."

What your body hears: "Surprise glucose spike incoming!"

Science Snapshot: *Frequent snacking raises insulin exposure, impairs fat oxidation, and leads to higher overall calorie intake (Perrigue et al., 2016).*

Translation: Every "healthy" snack is a metabolic hostage negotiation.

Snacking Criteria for Rebels

Requirement	Minimum Standard
Protein	≥10g
Net Carbs	≤5g
Fat	Optional but welcome
Real food	Not a fiber-wrapped candy bar

Rebel Snack #1 — Hard-Boiled Eggs with Olive Oil + Salt
Ingredients:
- 2 boiled eggs
- 1 tsp olive oil
- Pinch of salt and pepper

Macros: Net Carbs: 1g | Protein: 12g | Fat: 10g

Science Snapshot: *Eggs reduce ghrelin and increase satiety longer than cereal or toast (Vander Wal et al., 2005).*

Translation: The snack that punches hunger in the face.

Rebel Snack #2 — Tuna in Olive Oil Pouch
Ingredients:
- 1 pouch (2.6 oz) tuna in olive oil

Macros: Net Carbs: 0g | Protein: 18g | Fat: 6g

Science Snapshot: *Protein-only snacks improve glucose stability and reduce subsequent meal sizes (Westerterp-Plantenga et al., 2004).*

Translation: Emergency protein with swagger.

Rebel Snack #3 — Full-Fat Greek Yogurt + Chia
Ingredients:
- ½ cup plain Greek yogurt (5% fat)
- 1 tbsp chia seeds
- Optional: cinnamon, stevia

Macros: Net Carbs: 5g | Protein: 15g | Fat: 8g

Science Snapshot: *Fermented dairy improves insulin sensitivity and reduces waist circumference (Drouin-Chartier et al., 2016).*

Translation: Not all white stuff in a tub are lies.

Rebel Snack #4 — Beef Jerky (No Sugar)

Ingredients:

- 2 oz unsweetened beef jerky

Macros: Net Carbs: 2g | Protein: 20g | Fat: 7g

Science Snapshot: *Lean protein between meals suppresses appetite and flattens post-meal glycemic spikes (Leidy et al., 2007).*

Translation: Read the label. If it says "teriyaki glaze," back away slowly.

Rebel Snack #5 — Sardines with Mustard

Ingredients:

- ½ can sardines in water or olive oil
- 1 tsp mustard

Macros: Net Carbs: 0g | Protein: 16g | Fat: 11g

Science Snapshot: *Fish-based snacks suppress appetite longer than carb snacks and support glucose control (Uhe et al., 1992).*

Translation: Smelly? Yes. Smart? Also yes.

Rebel Snack #6 — Edamame Pods with Sea Salt

Ingredients:

- ½ cup steamed edamame pods
- Pinch sea salt

Macros: Net Carbs: 4g | Protein: 11g | Fat: 6g

Science Snapshot: *Soy protein improves satiety and lowers cholesterol markers in insulin-resistant adults (Anderson et al., 1995).*

Translation: A snack that crunches but doesn't spike.

Rebel Snack #7 — Turkey-Cucumber Roll-Ups

Ingredients:

- 3 slices deli turkey
- 6 thin cucumber sticks
- Optional: smear of mustard

Macros: Net Carbs: 2g | Protein: 16g | Fat: 4g

Science Snapshot: *Low-fat protein snacks reduce calorie intake over 24 hours (Chapelot et al., 2010).*

Translation: The opposite of a "snack bar."

Rebel Snack #8 — Protein Shake (No Fruit)

Ingredients:

- 1 scoop whey or plant-based protein
- ½ cup water or almond milk
- Ice, blend to taste

Macros: Net Carbs: 3g | Protein: 25g | Fat: 3g

Science Snapshot: *Protein shakes between meals reduce glucose variability and improve energy regulation (Wang et al., 2008).*

Translation: Liquid fuel, not smoothie cosplay.

Rebel Snack #9 — Tofu Cubes with Coconut Aminos

Ingredients:

- ½ cup firm tofu, cubed
- 1 tsp coconut aminos
- Pinch garlic powder

Macros: Net Carbs: 3g | Protein: 12g | Fat: 9g

Science Snapshot: *Plant protein sources like tofu provide insulin-moderating effects with complete amino acid profiles (Messina, 2010).*

Translation: Not every snack needs to crunch to be strategic.

Rebel Snack #10 — Celery with Nut Butter

Ingredients:

- 2 celery sticks
- 2 tbsp almond or peanut butter

Macros: Net Carbs: 4g | Protein: 6g | Fat: 16g

Science Snapshot: *Fat combined with fiber delays gastric emptying and slows glucose absorption (Wolever et al., 1991).*

Translation: Spoonfuls are not a serving. Apply with intent.

Rebel Snack #11 — Sardines on Zucchini Slices

Ingredients:

- ½ tin sardines
- 5–6 raw zucchini coins
- Paprika or chili powder

Macros: Net Carbs: 2g | Protein: 13g | Fat: 9g

Science Snapshot: *Sardines improve insulin sensitivity and provide omega-3s that reduce inflammation (Di Giuseppe et al., 2014).*

Translation: The smell is aggressive, but so is the science.

Rebel Snack #12 — Avocado + Lemon + Salt (Spoon Snack)

Ingredients:

- ½ avocado
- Squeeze of lemon juice
- Salt and pepper

Macros: Net Carbs: 6g | Protein: 2g | Fat: 15g

Science Snapshot: *Monounsaturated fat lowers postprandial glucose and enhances insulin sensitivity (Wang et al., 2015).*

Translation: No cracker required. Just a spoon.

Rebel Snack #13 — Roasted Seaweed + Boiled Egg

Ingredients:

- 1 boiled egg
- 1–2 roasted seaweed sheets

Macros: Net Carbs: 1g | Protein: 8g | Fat: 7g

Science Snapshot: *Seaweed compounds regulate carbohydrate metabolism and support glucose stability (Peng et al., 2015).*

Translation: Crunchy. Salty. Functional.

Rebel Snack #14 — Jerky + Pickles

Ingredients:

- 1 oz sugar-free beef or turkey jerky
- 2 dill pickle spears

Macros: Net Carbs: 4g | Protein: 14g | Fat: 7g

Science Snapshot: *Pairing protein with vinegar-containing foods (like pickles) may blunt glycemic response (Liljeberg & Björck, 1998).*

Translation: Carnivore snack with a fermented sidekick.

Rebel Snack #15 — Egg Bites (Prepped Ahead)

Ingredients:

- 2 egg bites (baked with eggs, spinach, feta)

Macros (per 2): Net Carbs: 3g | Protein: 14g | Fat: 11g

Science Snapshot: *Protein-rich mini-meals prevent blood sugar dips and reduce cravings later in the day (Jakubowicz et al., 2013).*

Translation: Yes, you can eat them cold. No, you don't need a sugary drink disguised as coffee.

When to Snack (and When to Just Wait)

Situation	Snack?
Pre-workout	Yes, if last meal was >3 hrs ago
Late dinner	Yes, if you're genuinely hungry and need protein
Mindless boredom	Absolutely not
Stress at work	Drink water. Take a lap. Stop blaming almonds.
After a low-carb meal	If built right, you shouldn't need one

Science Snapshot: *People snack out of habit, not hunger—resulting in excess intake and higher fasting glucose (Hartmann et al., 2013).*

Translation: Not hungry? Don't feed the glucose gremlins.

Exit Ramp

You're allowed to snack—but not like a toddler at a birthday party. Be tactical. Be fed, not fooled. Snack like you mean it, or don't snack at all.

Rebel Command

1. Hunger is not the only reason people eat. Don't trust your cravings—audit them.
2. Snacking is not a meal replacement. It's a biochemical Band-Aid.
3. If you do it, do it like a rebel: protein-forward, carb-controlled, purpose-driven.

CHAPTER 11
BEVERAGES THAT DON'T BETRAY YOU

What's in Your Cup Shouldn't Wreck Your Metabolism

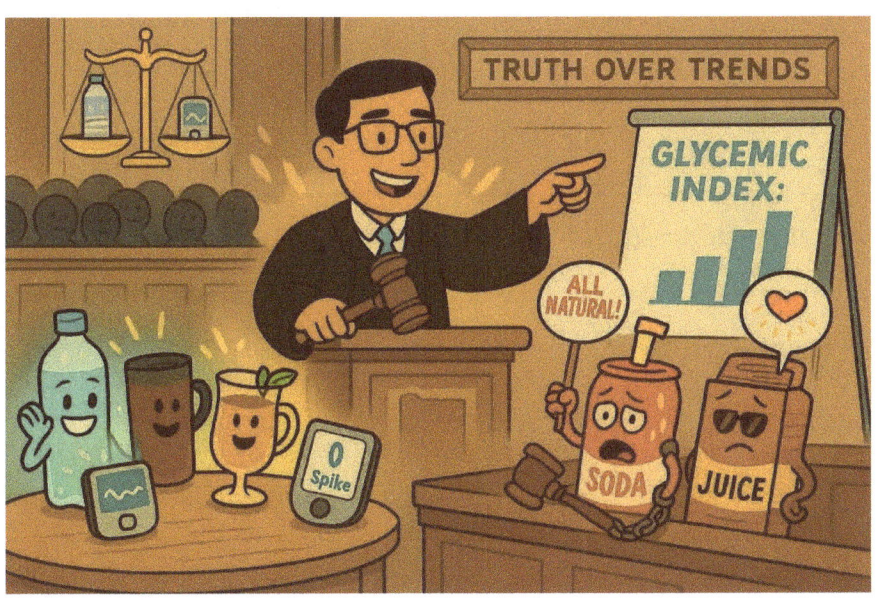

What You'll Learn

1. Why most drinks are dessert in disguise.
2. How to decode deceptive beverage labels and avoid liquid sabotage.
3. What you *can* drink freely, safely, and joyfully—without triggering a glucose spike or needing a support group.

Rebel Rallying Cry

Beverages are where most people blow their metabolism without chewing a single bite. If your drink has calories and a marketing team, assume it's guilty until proven otherwise.

The Beverage Betrayal — Some Usual Suspects

Drink	Hidden Threat
Fruit juice	Liquid fructose bomb with a health halo
Iced coffee drinks	Milkshakes with espresso
Sports drinks	Engineered for athletes—consumed by couch potatoes
Plant-based milk	Often contains added sugar, rice syrup, or pure nonsense
Flavored water	Usually "essence of glucose"
Kombucha	May have more sugar than soda (check the label!)

Science Snapshot: *Sugary drinks are the fastest way to spike insulin and contribute to fatty liver, even without weight gain (Stanhope et al., 2009).*

Translation: If your pancreas had a blacklist, liquid sugar would be on top.

Rebel Beverage Guidelines

Rule	Why It Matters
Zero added sugars	Prevent glucose spikes and insulin release
Minimal net carbs (≤2g)	Keeps fat oxidation humming
No artificial crap	Your liver's got enough to do
Electrolytes over energy drinks	Energy comes from real fuel, not taurine and fizz
Hydrate with intention	Thirst is not hunger. It's an unmet biological need.

Rebel Drinks You Can Count On

1. Water

Obvious? Yes. Done well? Rarely. Add lemon, cucumber, or mint to make it feel like a choice.

Why it wins: Zero calories, supports detox, curbs false hunger.

2. Mineral Water or Sparkling Water

Flavored? Only if it has no sweeteners.

Look for: Ingredients list with only water + natural essence.

Why it wins: Bubbles without betrayal.

3. Black Coffee

Add cinnamon or a dash of heavy cream if you must.

Why it wins: Caffeine boosts fat oxidation and suppresses appetite.

Science Snapshot: *Black coffee improves insulin sensitivity in the short term (Wedick et al., 2011).*

Translation: Coffee = thermogenic rebellion.

4. Unsweetened Herbal Tea

Chamomile, rooibos, peppermint—calm without chaos.

Why it wins: Warm, comforting, zero spike.

Bonus: May improve sleep, reduce stress.

5. Bone Broth (Unsalted or Homemade)

Protein in liquid form, ideal between meals.

Why it wins: Collagen, amino acids, electrolytes.

Science Snapshot: *Glycine supports insulin regulation and satiety (Cynober, 2002).*

Translation: Broth isn't just for grandmas. It's biochemical maintenance.

Rebel Add-Ons (Use With Caution)

Add-On	Verdict
Heavy cream (1–2 tbsp)	Fine in coffee—minimal carbs, adds satiety
Almond milk (unsweetened)	Acceptable—watch for gums, fillers
Electrolyte powders	Only if no added sugar or maltodextrin
Lemon juice	Great in water, supports liver function
Protein powder in drinks	Yes—but make sure it's not dessert cosplay

Top Beverage Betrayals (to Ditch Immediately)

Beverage	Reason to Nuke It
Smoothies with banana, date, mango	Fructose bombs with a blender's alibi
"Lite" sports drinks	Still spike blood sugar, often contain hidden sugars
Diet sodas	Artificial sweeteners may impair insulin sensitivity and gut microbiome *(Suez et al., 2014)*

Beverage	Reason to Nuke It
Kombucha (with >5g sugar)	Fermented doesn't mean free pass
Plant milks with rice/oat	They're basically drinkable carbs

Exit Ramp

If you wouldn't spoon sugar into your mouth, don't sip it out of a straw. Your drinks should hydrate you, fuel you, or chill you out—not destabilize your glucose and fry your liver.

Rebel Command

1. If it's sweet and liquid, it's probably spiking you.
2. Read the label like your metabolism depends on it—because it does.
3. Water isn't boring. Metabolic chaos is.

CHAPTER 12
DIPS, DRESSINGS, AND SAUCES THAT WON'T TAKE YOU DOWN

Flavor Without the Spike

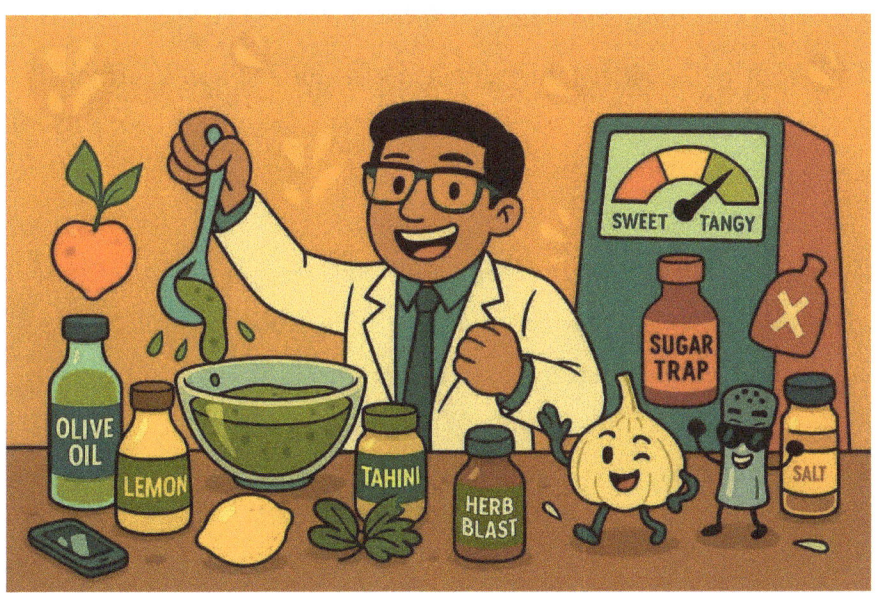

What You'll Learn

1. Why most store-bought condiments are sugar traps wearing organic labels.
2. How to build flavor bombs that upgrade your meals without detonating your glucose.
3. 15 dips, dressings, and sauces that turn basic food into metabolic firepower.

Rebel Rallying Cry

Food shouldn't be bland just because your pancreas is picky. But if your "healthy" salad dressing has 8 grams of sugar per tablespoon, you didn't eat a salad—you ate dessert on a leaf. Welcome to the flavor revolution—no glucose sabotage required.

The Hidden Saboteurs in Your Fridge Door

That bottle of honey mustard? Syrup in disguise.

Your favorite "balsamic vinaigrette"? A slow-motion insulin grenade.

Ketchup? Sugar in a red coat.

Science Snapshot: *Most commercial condiments contain hidden sugars and refined oils that trigger inflammation and elevate post-meal glucose—even in small servings (Lustig et al., 2012).*

Translation: If your condiment has a paragraph of ingredients and ends in "-ose," it's not a sauce—it's a setback.

Rebel Flavor Commandments

Commandment	Why It Matters
Real fat is your friend	Satiety + flavor + stable glucose
Sugar = betrayal	Even "just a touch" adds up fast
Read the label (then mock it)	"Serving size: 1 tsp" is marketing fiction

Dips, Dressings, and Sauces That Won't Take You Down

Commandment	Why It Matters
Acid is underrated	Vinegar + citrus = blood sugar control + zing
Herbs > hype	Fresh, dried, ground—they make you forget sugar

Drips, Dressing, Sauces (DDS) #1 — Rebel Ranch
Ingredients:
- ½ cup full-fat Greek yogurt
- 2 tbsp mayo (avocado or olive oil-based)
- 1 tsp garlic powder, 1 tsp onion powder
- 1 tsp dried dill, salt, pepper
- Splash of lemon juice

Macros: Net Carbs: 2g | Fat: 14g | Protein: 4g

Science Snapshot: *Full-fat dairy improves insulin sensitivity and promotes satiety (Drouin-Chartier et al., 2016).*

Translation: It's ranch. Without the sugar. Without the shame.

DDS #2 — Avocado-Lime Smash
Ingredients:
- 1 ripe avocado
- Juice of ½ lime
- Garlic, cumin, chili flakes
- Salt to taste

Macros: Net Carbs: 4g | Fat: 15g | Protein: 2g

Science Snapshot: *Avocados reduce postprandial glucose and insulin spikes (Wang et al., 2015).*

Translation: Guac it out—just skip the chips.

DDS #3 — Spicy Tahini Drizzle
Ingredients

- 2 tbsp tahini
- 1 tbsp lemon juice
- 1 tsp olive oil
- Pinch of cayenne
- Warm water to thin

Macros: Net Carbs: 2g | Fat: 12g | Protein: 3g

Science Snapshot: *Sesame seed fat improves lipid profiles and metabolic flexibility (Moazzami et al., 2009).*

Translation: Your salad's new best friend, minus the insulin tax.

DDS #4 — No-Sugar Ketchup
Ingredients:

- ¼ cup tomato paste
- 2 tbsp apple cider vinegar
- ½ tsp garlic powder
- Pinch of clove, salt, and allulose or monk fruit to taste

Macros: Net Carbs: 3g | Fat: 0g | Protein: 1g

Science Snapshot: *Commercial ketchup can contain up to 1 tsp sugar per tablespoon (FDA, 2020).*

Translation: The fries may be fake, but your ketchup doesn't have to be.

DDS #5 — Zesty Green Goddess
Ingredients:
- ½ avocado
- Handful of parsley and cilantro
- 1 tbsp lemon juice
- 1 tbsp olive oil
- 2 tbsp water
- Salt, garlic

Macros: Net Carbs: 3g | Fat: 13g | Protein: 2g

Science Snapshot: *Fresh herbs contain polyphenols that improve metabolic markers (Pérez-Jiménez et al., 2010).*

Translation: Green magic for meat, veg, or spooning straight from the jar.

DDS #6 — Rebel Aioli
Ingredients:
- 2 tbsp avocado oil mayo
- 1 clove minced garlic
- ½ tsp lemon juice
- Salt, smoked paprika

Macros: Net Carbs: 1g | Fat: 20g | Protein: 1g

Science Snapshot: *Garlic reduces blood pressure and improves fasting glucose (Ried et al., 2008).*

Translation: It's mayo—but tactical.

DDS #7 — Cauli-Hummus
Ingredients:
- 1 cup steamed cauliflower
- 1 tbsp tahini
- 1 clove garlic
- 1 tbsp lemon juice
- Salt, cumin

Macros: Net Carbs: 5g | Fat: 6g | Protein: 3g

Science Snapshot: *Cauliflower provides fiber and micronutrients without causing the glucose elevations often seen with legumes like lentils or chickpeas, especially in insulin-resistant individuals (Wolever & Jenkins, 1986).*

Translation: Hummus, but without the chickpea drama.

DDS #8 — Yogurt-Dill Dip
Ingredients:
- ½ cup full-fat Greek yogurt
- 1 tbsp chopped fresh dill
- 1 tsp lemon juice
- Salt, garlic powder

Macros: Net Carbs: 2g | Fat: 4g | Protein: 7g

Science Snapshot: *Yogurt with herbs supports gut flora and glycemic control (Marco et al., 2017).*

Translation: It's tzatziki's smug cousin.

DDS #9 — Basil-Walnut Pesto

Ingredients:

- 1 cup fresh basil
- ¼ cup walnuts
- 2 tbsp olive oil
- 1 clove garlic
- Salt

Macros: Net Carbs: 3g | Fat: 15g | Protein: 3g

Science Snapshot: *Pesto's healthy fats and polyphenols improve satiety and reduce oxidative stress (Mozaffarian et al., 2010).*

Translation: Pasta's gone. Pesto stayed.

DDS #10 — Spicy Peanut Sauce

Ingredients:

- 2 tbsp natural peanut butter
- 1 tbsp coconut aminos
- 1 tsp rice vinegar
- Dash of chili flakes, garlic

Macros: Net Carbs: 4g | Fat: 14g | Protein: 6g

Science Snapshot: *Peanut butter lowers post-meal glucose when combined with protein and fiber (Johnston et al., 2002).*

Translation: Wok-tossed joy without the insulin aftermath.

DDS #11 — Creamy Cumin Dressing

Ingredients:

- 2 tbsp olive oil
- 1 tbsp lime juice
- 1 tsp ground cumin
- Salt, garlic powder

Macros: Net Carbs: 1g | Fat: 14g | Protein: 0g

Science Snapshot: *Cumin may reduce fasting glucose and lipid markers (Nematy et al., 2013).*

Translation: Spicy, savory, and insulin-approved.

DDS #12 — Smoky Eggplant Dip (Baba Sans-nouche)

Ingredients:

- 1 roasted eggplant
- 1 tbsp tahini
- 1 tsp lemon juice
- Garlic, olive oil, salt

Macros: Net Carbs: 5g | Fat: 10g | Protein: 2g

Science Snapshot: *Eggplant polyphenols improve glucose metabolism (Kwon et al., 2008).*

Translation: Dip that doesn't dip your energy.

DDS #13 — Dijon Vinaigrette

Ingredients:

- 2 tbsp olive oil
- 1 tsp Dijon mustard
- 1 tbsp apple cider vinegar
- Salt, pepper, herbs

Macros: Net Carbs: 1g | Fat: 14g | Protein: 0g

Science Snapshot: *Vinegar reduces post-meal glucose spikes when consumed with carbs (Johnston et al., 2004).*

Translation: This dressing earns its place on your plate.

DDS #14 — Coconut-Curry Sauce

Ingredients:

- ¼ cup full-fat coconut milk
- ½ tsp curry powder
- ¼ tsp turmeric
- Salt, lime juice

Macros: Net Carbs: 3g | Fat: 12g | Protein: 1g

Science Snapshot: *MCTs in coconut improve fat metabolism and reduce insulin spikes (St-Onge et al., 2003).*

Translation: Tropical. Tactical. Tastebud-approved.

DDS #15 — Sun-Dried Tomato Tapenade

Ingredients:

- ¼ cup sun-dried tomatoes (no sugar added)
- 1 tbsp olive oil
- Garlic, herbs, salt

Macros: Net Carbs: 4g | Fat: 10g | Protein: 2g

Science Snapshot: *Lycopene in tomatoes supports insulin sensitivity and vascular health (Li et al., 2014).*

Translation: Your meatballs just leveled up.

Red Flag Sauces (That Pretend to Be Healthy)

Label Claim	Reality Check
"Honey Mustard"	That's just sugar and PR
"Balsamic Glaze"	Sugar syrup with a diploma
"Fat-Free Caesar"	Carbs + MSG cocktail

Label Claim	Reality Check
"Sweet Chili Sauce"	Dessert in a dipping bowl
"Keto BBQ"	Still spikes if maltitol shows up

Exit Ramp

Flavor is not the enemy. Sugar sneaking in through your sauce is. These dips, dressings, and sauces let you eat boldly—without spiking, crashing, or compromising. Your food just went from compliant to combat-ready.

Rebel Command

1. If your sauce comes with a glucose bill, cancel it.
2. Fat + acid + herbs = flavor with a function.
3. Label-free, sugar-free, guilt-free—dip like you mean it.

PART III:
STRATEGY, SURVIVAL, AND SCIENCE

CHAPTER 13
FLAVOR SCIENCE FOR REBELS

*How to Hack Your Taste Buds, Retrain Cravings,
and Dethrone the Snack Food Industry*

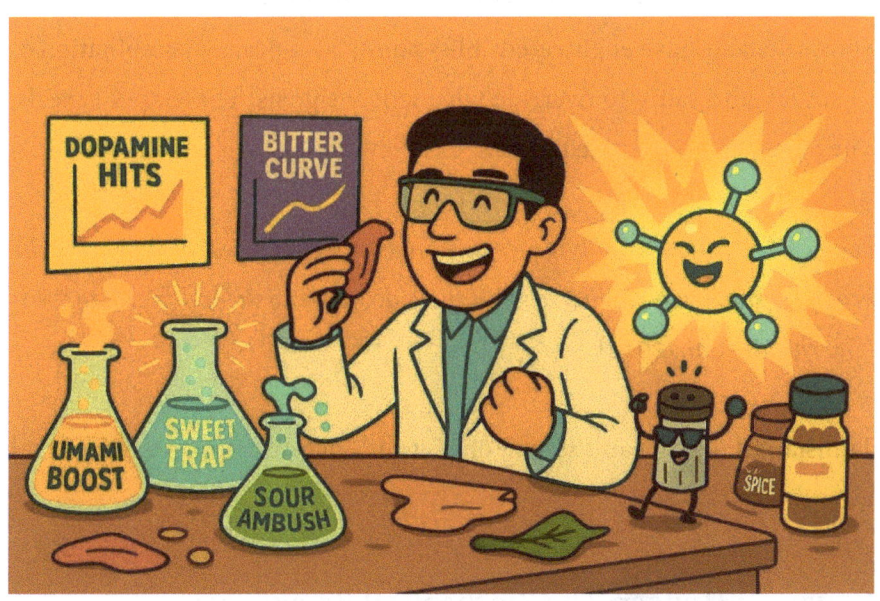

What You'll Learn

1. Why your cravings are manufactured—not moral failings.
2. The neurobiology of flavor addiction (a.k.a. why chips make you eat the whole bag).
3. How to reset your taste buds, dominate your cravings, and fall in love with real food again.

Rebel Rallying Cry

If you've ever found yourself elbow-deep in a bag of "healthy" crackers while swearing it's the last one, you've already met the enemy. And the enemy has a lab coat, a spreadsheet, and a flavor algorithm. This is not a battle of willpower. It's a biochemical hostage situation—and it's time to negotiate your release.

The Flavor Matrix Was Designed to Break You

Food scientists have engineered "bliss points"—a precise combination of sugar, fat, and salt—to override your satiety signals. These aren't meals. They're edible dopamine triggers.

Science Snapshot: *Highly processed foods activate reward centers in the brain the same way addictive substances do, making them difficult to resist (Gearhardt et al., 2011).*

Translation: If you can't stop at one bite, it's because it was designed that way.

Craving ≠ Hunger: The Biochemical Breakdown

Signal	Meaning	Typical Trigger
True hunger	Body needs fuel	Time since last protein-rich meal
Craving	Brain wants a reward	Stress, habit, dopamine lull

Signal	Meaning	Typical Trigger
Habitual urge	Mental association	Commercials, location, boredom
Blood sugar crash	Desperation	High-carb meal 1–2 hours ago

Solution? Stabilize glucose, eat real food, and give your palate a chance to remember what food is *supposed* to taste like.

How to Reset Your Palate (and Take Down the Flavor Cartel)

Step 1 — Cut the Dopamine Supply Chain

Minimize ultra-processed foods, artificial sweeteners, and taste "hacks" that mimic sugar. This reduces the over-stimulation that makes whole foods taste "bland" by comparison.

Step 2 — Reintroduce Real Flavors

Retrain your taste buds with herbs, spices, acidity, and natural bitterness. Use salt with intention—not as camouflage.

Step 3 — Prioritize Texture and Contrast

Satiety increases with variety in texture and temperature—crunchy greens with warm protein, crispy nuts with creamy dips.

Step 4 — Embrace the Bitter and the Sour

Bitterness signals micronutrients. Sourness stimulates digestion. Retrain your palate to recognize these flavors as *real food markers*, not red flags.

Flavor-Building Blocks for Rebels

Flavor Type	Real Examples	Why It Helps
Umami	Mushrooms, tomatoes, meat, miso	Signals protein, promotes satiety
Sour	Lemon, vinegar, fermented foods	Enhances digestion and flavor clarity
Bitter	Arugula, kale, cocoa, coffee	Slows eating speed and overconsumption
Salty	Sea salt, olives, feta	Enhances natural flavor—use sparingly
Fatty	Olive oil, avocado, coconut, tahini	Increases satiety and food satisfaction
Spicy	Ginger, black pepper, chili flakes	Increases metabolic rate, adds complexity

Rebel Flavor Hacks to Crush Cravings Without Glucose Drama

- **Roast your veggies** with salt and oil to caramelize natural sugars.
- **Add acid** (lemon, vinegar) to finish protein dishes—balances fat and makes you want less.
- **Use a spice blend** (like Za'atar, Berbere, or curry powder) to turn boring into bold.
- **Fat-fiber-protein trifecta** in one bite = satiety amplifier.
- **Don't forget texture**: crunch + creaminess = crave-able without carbs.

Manufactured Cravings: Know Your Triggers

Situation	Engineered Food That Fills the Gap (But Sabotages You)	Rebel Upgrade
Afternoon crash	Protein bar with "natural sugars"	Hard-boiled eggs + olive oil
Post-dinner urge	"Healthy" frozen yogurt	Chia custard or cocoa avocado mousse
PMS or stress binge	Chocolate bars, crackers	Dark chocolate + almonds or Greek yogurt + cocoa
"I'm being good" celebration	Granola bars, oat cookies	Almond-coconut bites or lemon cheesecake fat bombs

Science Snapshot: *Taste buds regenerate every 10–14 days. If you cut out hyper-palatable foods for two weeks, your taste recalibrates—making real food satisfying again (Stewart et al., 2020).*

Translation: Your body isn't addicted to flavor. It's addicted to a hijacked version of it. Time to uninstall the malware.

Exit Ramp

Food isn't supposed to be addictive. It's supposed to be satisfying. You're not weak—you've been neurologically manipulated. But the flavor matrix can be rewritten. And you're the one holding the pen (and the seasoning).

Rebel Command

1. Flavor engineering is real—and reversible.
2. Cravings don't mean you're broken. They mean you're programmable.
3. Real food isn't boring. Your taste buds have just been hacked. Time to reboot.

CHAPTER 14
GROCERY STORE GUERRILLA TACTICS

Shop Like a Metabolic Insurgent in a World
That Wants You Addicted to Snack Cakes

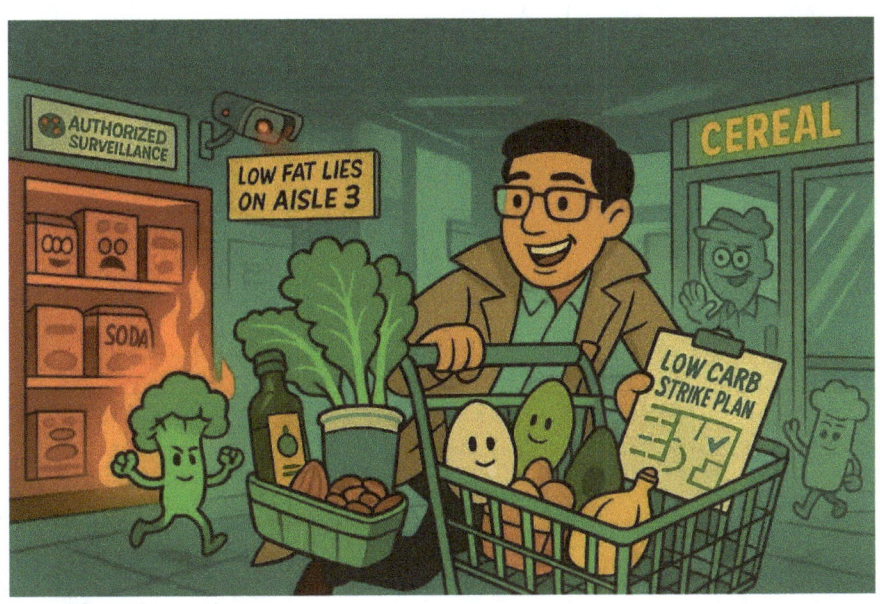

What You'll Learn

1. How to navigate the grocery store like a rebel, not a lab rat.
2. How to decode labels, dodge traps, and fill your cart with glucose-slaying ingredients.
3. Why the center aisles are booby-trapped—and how to escape with your pancreas intact.

Rebel Rallying Cry

The modern grocery store is a battlefield disguised as a convenience. Every aisle is designed to optimize *your surrender*—to sugar, snacks, fake health claims, and impulse buys. But you're not here to browse. You're here to strategize. This is tactical grocery acquisition, not a Sunday stroll.

The Store is Rigged Against You—Let's Break It Down:

Zone	What It Sells	Why It's Dangerous
End caps	"Deals" on processed foods	Designed to trigger impulse buys
Center aisles	Cereal, chips, "bars"	High-margin, hyper-palatable, blood sugar bombs
Checkout lane	Candy, soda, gum	One last chance to spike your insulin
Front of store	"Health" drinks, smoothies, granola	Where lies go to be packaged in green labels

Science Snapshot: *Product placement increases calorie and sugar purchases even in health-conscious shoppers (Cohen & Babey, 2012).*

Translation: The supermarket is not your friend. It's a glucose trap with air conditioning.

The Rebel Grocery War Plan

1. Perimeter First, Center Last (If At All)

The good stuff lives on the edges—produce, meat, eggs, dairy, frozen veg. Center aisles are mostly entertainment food in edible form.

2. List or Die

If you go in without a list, you're going in unarmed. Even rebels need a plan.

3. Read the Label Like a Spy, Not a Tourist

- Look past "keto," "natural," and "gluten-free."
- Go straight to the *ingredients list* and *net carbs*.
- If sugar or starch is in the top 5, it's a no.

Ingredient Code Words That Mean "Sugar"

What It Says	What It Means
Brown rice syrup	Liquid sugar with a hat on
Organic cane juice	Sugar with a clean conscience
Agave nectar	A fructose bomb with a flower name
Maltodextrin	Glucose rocket fuel
Fruit concentrate	Juice pretending it's whole fruit
Evaporated cane syrup	Still syrup. Still sugar.

Rebel Shopping List: Low-Carb, High-Impact Staples

Proteins
- Eggs
- Chicken thighs, drumsticks
- Ground turkey, beef, lamb
- Tofu, tempeh
- Sardines, salmon, shrimp
- Greek yogurt (full-fat, unsweetened)

Vegetables
- Spinach, kale, arugula
- Cauliflower, broccoli, zucchini
- Mushrooms, peppers, cucumbers
- Frozen veg (no sauces)

Fats & Condiments
- Olive oil, avocado oil, coconut oil
- Avocados
- Nuts, seeds (almonds, chia, flax)
- Tahini, nut butters (no sugar added)
- Mustard, vinegar, salsa, hot sauce
- Full-fat cheeses (goat, feta, cheddar)

Extras
- Chia seeds, psyllium husk
- Almond flour, coconut flour
- Stevia, erythritol, monk fruit
- Dark chocolate (85%+)
- Protein powders (whey, pea, collagen)

Label Reading 101: The Rebel Audit Checklist

Ask yourself:

- Are total net carbs under 5g per serving?
- Is protein ≥10g (if it claims to be high-protein)?
- Is fat coming from real sources (nuts, oils, eggs)?
- Are there fewer than 10 ingredients?
- Can I pronounce everything without a PhD in food chemistry?

If not: it goes back on the shelf.

Rebel Warning Signs on "Health" Foods

Label Claim	Actual Meaning
Keto-friendly	Still needs a label check. Could be maltitol-laced betrayal.
Gluten-free	Doesn't mean low-carb. Could be rice flour and sugar grenades.
Plant-based	Often = starch-based + syrup.
Low-fat	Almost always = high-sugar.
Vegan cookies	Still cookies. Still glucose drama.

Exit Ramp

Your grocery cart is your front line. You either leave that store equipped for rebellion—or set up to fail by snack propaganda. Load your cart with food that fuels, not foods that manipulate. Be the one person in line whose groceries make sense.

Rebel Command

1. The grocery store is a behavioral lab with freezers. Don't be the rat.
2. Read labels like you're disarming a glucose bomb—because you are.
3. You're not shopping for fun. You're shopping to win.

CHAPTER 15
KITCHEN SETUP FOR THE BLOOD SUGAR BATTLE

Tools, Tricks, and Tactical Appliances for Low-Carb Combat

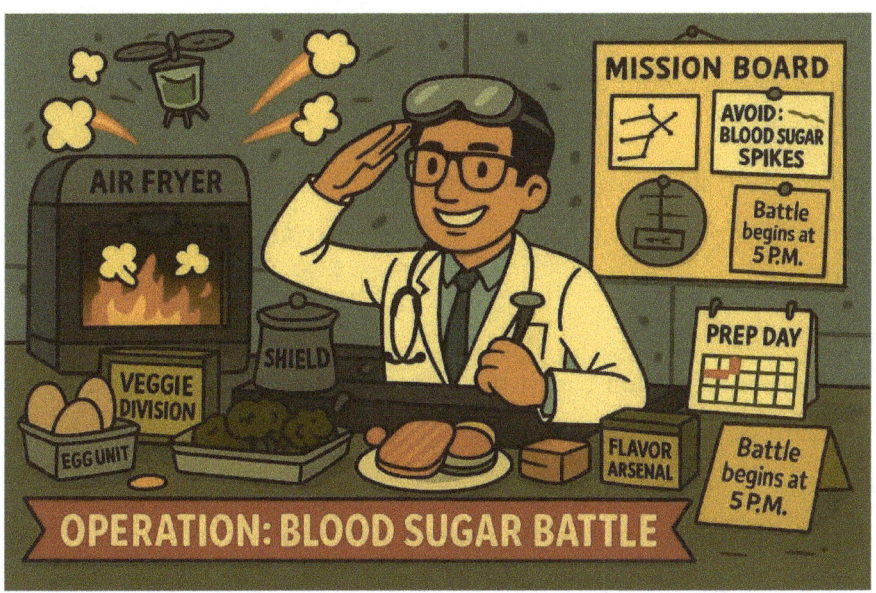

What You'll Learn

1. How to turn your kitchen into a metabolic war room—not a sabotage zone.
2. What to keep, what to ditch, and what to upgrade.
3. How to organize your tools, pantry, and prep flow so that success becomes automatic and sabotage becomes inconvenient.

Rebel Rallying Cry

You can't win a battle with a butter knife. Your kitchen shouldn't be a passive backdrop—it should be a fortified command center designed to make rebellion easy and blood sugar spikes nearly impossible.

If Your Kitchen Looks Like a Snack Bar, You'll Eat Like a Snack Bar

Your kitchen setup influences your choices more than your willpower. If the cereal is front and center and the olive oil is behind six dusty cans of cranberry sauce, your environment is not your ally.

Science Snapshot: *People who keep visible fruit or healthy proteins on counters weigh less than those who keep cereal, soda, or baked goods visible (Wansink, 2016).*

Translation: You don't eat what's "good." You eat what's nearby. So make the good stuff unavoidable.

The 5 Commandments of a Rebel Kitchen

Commandment	Strategy
1. Visibility = Destiny	Keep protein, veg, and healthy fats in sight.
2. Inconvenience the Sabotage	Junk food should be in the basement—or better, the garbage.

Commandment	Strategy
3. Prep Trumps Willpower	Have proteins, chopped veg, and sauces ready before hunger hits.
4. Equip for Simplicity	If your blender requires tech support to operate, it's the wrong tool.
5. Label with Purpose	Containers should scream "fuel," not "snack me."

Appliances That Earn Their Counter Space

Tool	Why It's Rebel-Approved
Air fryer	Crisps veg and proteins fast, no added carbs.
Pressure cooker (e.g., Instant Pot)	Batch-cooks proteins and stews in under an hour.
Blender (basic, not barista-grade)	Makes chia pudding, sauces, or protein drinks—fast.
Measuring spoons/cups	For when your "just a splash" becomes 5 tablespoons of almond butter.
Good nonstick or cast iron pan	You'll be cooking. Often. Don't fight your cookware.
Glass containers with lids	Store prepped food visibly and neatly. Not a plastic tomb of mystery meals.

The Rebel Pantry: No Rations, No Excuses

Dry Goods & Staples

- Almond flour, coconut flour
- Chia seeds, flaxseed, psyllium
- Stevia, monk fruit, erythritol
- Canned tuna, sardines, salmon
- Vinegars (apple cider, balsamic)
- Herbs and spices (cumin, turmeric, paprika, garlic powder)
- Salt (kosher, sea, Himalayan)

Fats

- Olive oil, avocado oil
- Coconut oil
- Ghee
- Nut butters (no sugar added)

Fridge Staples

- Eggs
- Full-fat yogurt
- Leafy greens
- Prepped veggies
- Lemon juice
- Proteins (thawed and ready to go)

Freezer Essentials

- Frozen cauliflower, spinach, zucchini
- Ground meats, fish portions
- Chopped onions and stir-fry blends (no sauces)
- Ice trays for broth, herbs, or lemon juice cubes

Fridge Setup for Maximum Metabolic Wins

- Top Shelf — Prepped proteins, meals in glass containers
- Middle — Eggs, yogurt, leafy greens
- Bottom drawer — Washed veggies, visible, ready-to-eat
- Door — Condiments that support flavor without sugar
- Back of fridge — Nothing you want to eat. Keep it clean.

Rebel Prep Tactics for the Time-Strapped

- **Prep once, eat thrice:** Cook protein in batches—grill six chicken thighs, not one.
- **Veggie jar system:** Keep cut cucumbers, bell peppers, celery in glass jars for grab-and-crunch.
- **Sauce it smart:** One jar of tahini + lemon + garlic = dressing, dip, and marinade.
- **Chop with purpose:** When you're already cutting a bell pepper, do three. Store the rest.

Science Snapshot: *People who prep meals in advance eat significantly fewer calories and carbs (Berardy et al., 2019).*

Translation: Meal prep isn't extra work. It's metabolic insurance.

Exit Ramp

Your kitchen is either a launch pad or a liability. If you don't organize it like your health depends on it, it will betray you the minute you're tired, stressed, or rushed. Make rebellion the easy choice—by design.

Rebel Command

1. The war for your blood sugar is won in the kitchen—before you're hungry.
2. Prep beats willpower. Visibility beats intention.
3. Equip like a rebel. Shop like a scientist. Cook like you mean it.

CHAPTER 16
EXERCISE FOR PEOPLE WHO'D RATHER NAP

*Blood Sugar, Movement, and Why You Don't Need
a Gym to Win This War*

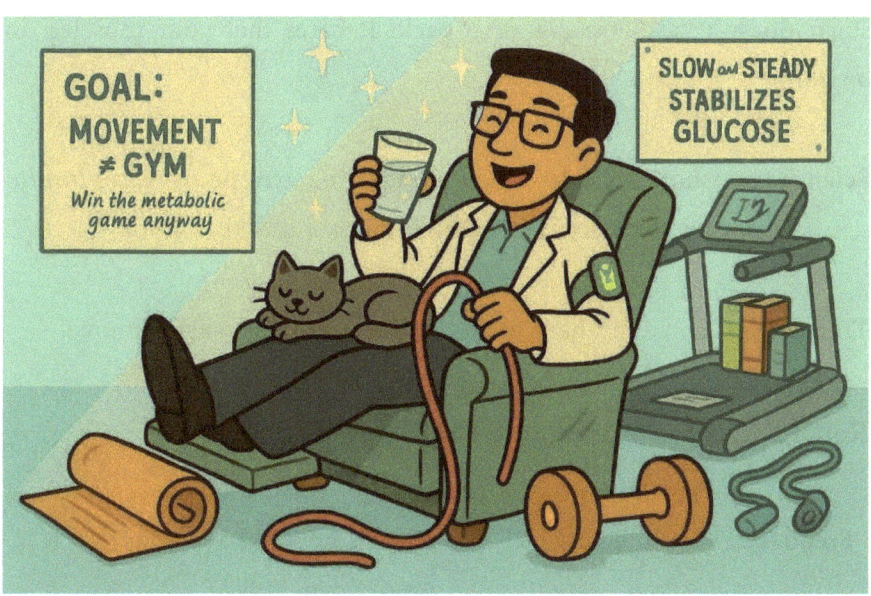

What You'll Learn

1. Why exercise matters more for blood sugar than weight loss.
2. How even tiny, intentional movements have outsized metabolic impact.
3. Simple, rebel-approved ways to build activity into your life—no gym, guilt, or supportive stretch-wear required.

Rebel Rallying Cry

You don't have to become an athlete. You don't have to enjoy burpees. You don't even have to sweat (though you might). You just need to move like someone who doesn't want their glucose wrecking their mitochondria. This isn't about sculpted abs. It's about metabolic mutiny.

The Exercise Illusion

The fitness industry lied to you. It made you think if you couldn't commit to an hour-long bootcamp class, it wasn't worth doing. That's false. Blood sugar doesn't care about your 6-pack. It cares that your muscles do *anything*.

Science Snapshot: *A single session of moderate exercise increases insulin sensitivity for up to 48 hours (Hawley & Lessard, 2008).*

Translation: You don't have to be shredded. You just have to move.

Rebel Rules for Movement That Works

Principle	What It Means
Frequency over intensity	10-minute walks > 1-hour weekly gym guilt
Post-meal movement > fasting HIIT	Your muscles are sugar sinks—use them after eating
Consistency wins	Movement snacks beat heroic marathons followed by 6-day couch comas

Principle	What It Means
Strength > scale	Build muscle, not misery
Do what you'll actually do	Dance counts. So does walking your dog. Rebellion is flexible.

Top Rebel Exercises That Smash Glucose (No Gym Required)

1. Post-Meal Walks (10–20 min)

Why it works: Moves glucose out of blood and into muscle like insulin's wingman.

Science Snapshot: *Walking after meals reduces postprandial glucose by 22% (Colberg et al., 2009).*

Translation: Walk off dinner. Literally.

2. Bodyweight Squats

Why it works: Quads are huge glucose-burning engines.
How to: Sit back into an imaginary chair. Rise. Repeat.

Set: 2–3 sets of 10–20 reps during TV commercials.

3. Wall Pushups

Why it works: Upper body strength, minimal intimidation.
How to: Hands on a wall, lean forward, push.

Set: 2 sets of 10–15, post-breakfast or lunch.

4. Kitchen Counter Calf Raises

Why it works: Builds stability, works big muscle groups while making coffee.

How to: Raise heels slowly. Hold. Lower with control.

Set: 3 sets of 15. Bonus: burns off grocery-store rage.

5. Resistance Band Rows

Why it works: Activates back, arms, and core—all with inexpensive rubber.

How to: Anchor band to doorknob. Pull like you're rowing away from glucose.

Movement Snacks: The Rebel Energy Boost

Time	Movement	Benefit
Morning	5 min stretch + squats	Wake up muscle, suppress glucose rise from breakfast
After meals	10 min walk	Clear blood glucose spike
Midday slump	3 min of shadowboxing or dancing	Dopamine + energy reset
Pre-bed	Gentle yoga or slow squats	Improve insulin sensitivity overnight

"I Don't Have Time" vs. Tactical Movement

Excuse	Rebel Response
"I'm too busy"	5 minutes = 288 minutes/month. You're not too busy.
"I don't like gyms"	Great. Your living room is fine.
"I'm too tired"	Movement *makes* energy. It's fuel, not a drain.
"I don't know what to do"	See above. Start with walking. No certification required.

Why Muscle Is Your Metabolic Bodyguard

Muscle isn't just for vanity. It's an active tissue that clears blood sugar, burns fat, and produces anti-inflammatory molecules. Lose muscle, lose metabolic power.

Science Snapshot: *Higher muscle mass is associated with better glucose regulation and reduced risk of Type 2 diabetes—even in people with higher BMI (Srikanthan & Karlamangla, 2011).*

Translation: You don't need less weight. You need more muscle.

Exit Ramp

You don't need a gym. You don't need a program. You just need to move—often, intentionally, and joyfully. Motion is rebellion. Stillness is surrender. Pick your side.

Rebel Command

1. Your muscles are glucose sponges. Use them.
2. Short, frequent movement trumps heroic overexertion.
3. If your body can move, it must move. Not for vanity—for victory.

CHAPTER 17
REBEL PSYCHOLOGY

*Why Your Brain Sabotages Your Progress
and How to Outsmart It with Humor, Grit, and Science*

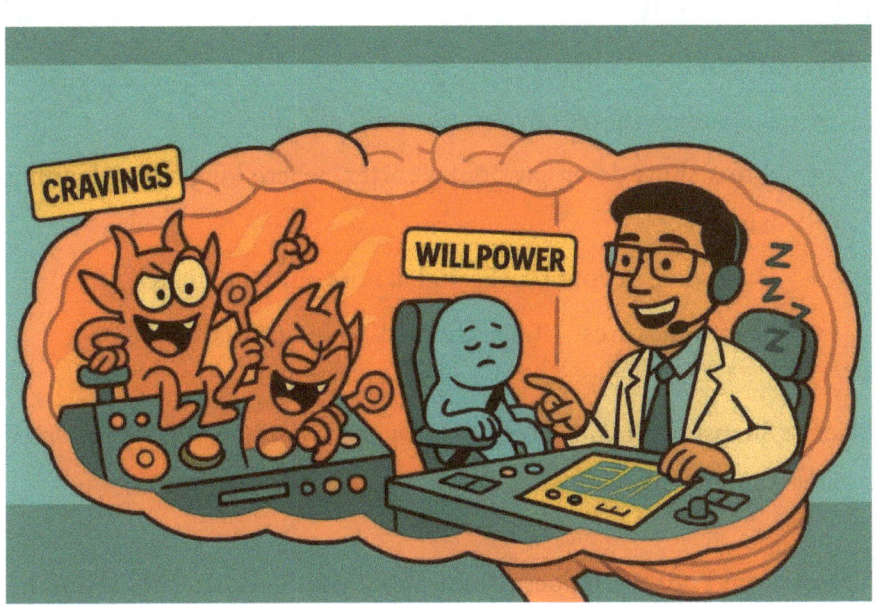

What You'll Learn

1. Why your brain prefers chips to discipline—and how to fix that.
2. The science behind habit formation, motivation, and failure cycles.
3. Mental hacks to stay on track without needing monk-level willpower.

Rebel Rallying Cry

This isn't just about what's on your plate. It's about what's in your head. You're not lazy. You're human. The modern world is designed to make you tired, distracted, and hungry for convenience. But we're not here to survive it. We're here to break it.

The Brain's Programming Is Not Your Fault—But It Is Your Job to Rewrite It

Why You Sabotage Yourself

- Dopamine chases novelty, not consistency.
- Stress shuts down prefrontal cortex, where long-term planning happens.
- Habits live in your basal ganglia, not your logic center.
- Shame backfires—it fuels reward-seeking, not discipline.

Science Snapshot: *Habits form not through motivation, but repetition in a stable context (Wood & Neal, 2007).*

Translation: Your brain doesn't care about your goals. It cares about the path of least resistance.

Mental Roadblocks (and Rebel Workarounds)

Mental Trap	Why It Happens	Rebel Fix
"I blew it" spiral	Perfectionist trap	Use the phrase: "One bad meal doesn't erase the revolution"

Mental Trap	Why It Happens	Rebel Fix
All-or-nothing	Brain likes binary	Reframe: "Next bite, next choice, next win"
"I deserve this" eating	Emotional reward system	Find non-food wins: walks, books, texts, rebellion playlists
Habitual grazing	Cue-based eating	Change the cue. Move. Sip water. Reroute the urge.
Shame storm	Brain thinks punishment = control	Radical self-respect is more effective than self-loathing

How to Build a Rebel Mindset

1. Ditch Willpower. Install Systems.

- Keep defaults rebel-friendly (no bread-basket on the table, pre-cut veggies visible).
- Automate meals you like and trust.
- Batch-cook like your life depends on it—because metabolically, it does.

2. Reframe "Setbacks" as Data

- Ate the cookie? Cool. Why?
- Stress? Poor prep? Shame? Learn and adjust. Rebels aren't perfect—they're iterative.

3. Habit Stack Like a Ninja

Attach a new behavior to a current one.

- After brushing teeth → take electrolytes.
- After dinner → walk 10 minutes.
- During coffee → plan meals.

Science Snapshot: *Habits stick when tied to identity, not willpower (Duhigg, 2012; Clear, 2018).*

Translation: You don't "try" to be a rebel. You are one. Now act like it.

4. Use Your Brain Against Itself

- Make the "bad" choice inconvenient (snacks in attic = no snacks).
- Make the "good" choice frictionless (meal prep > fridge chaos).
- Visual cues beat inner lectures (post-it notes > guilt spiral).

Rebel Affirmations That Actually Work

"I don't eat that."
"I fuel like a fighter, not a victim."
"I don't need perfect. I need persistent."
"This is who I am now—not who I used to be."

Read them out loud. Stick them on your fridge. Tattoo them on your glucose monitor.

The Inner Critic Is Loud. Make the Rebel Louder.

Your brain will try to whisper:

- "You're behind."
- "You're failing."
- "This is too hard."

But you can answer louder:
- "I don't need perfect. I need next."
- "Today is not yesterday."
- "Metabolic freedom tastes better than sabotage."

Exit Ramp

The war is not just in the pantry. It's in your head. But your brain is reprogrammable. Neuro-plasticity is your ally. Humor is your fuel. Grit is your superpower. You're not losing. You're learning. Keep going.

Rebel Command

1. Your brain wants dopamine, not discipline. Use that knowledge against it.
2. Systems beat willpower. Identity beats motivation.
3. You're not here for perfect. You're here for power.

CHAPTER 18
WHEN THE WORLD PUSHES BACK

Social Pressure, Cultural Resistance, and Tactical Defiance

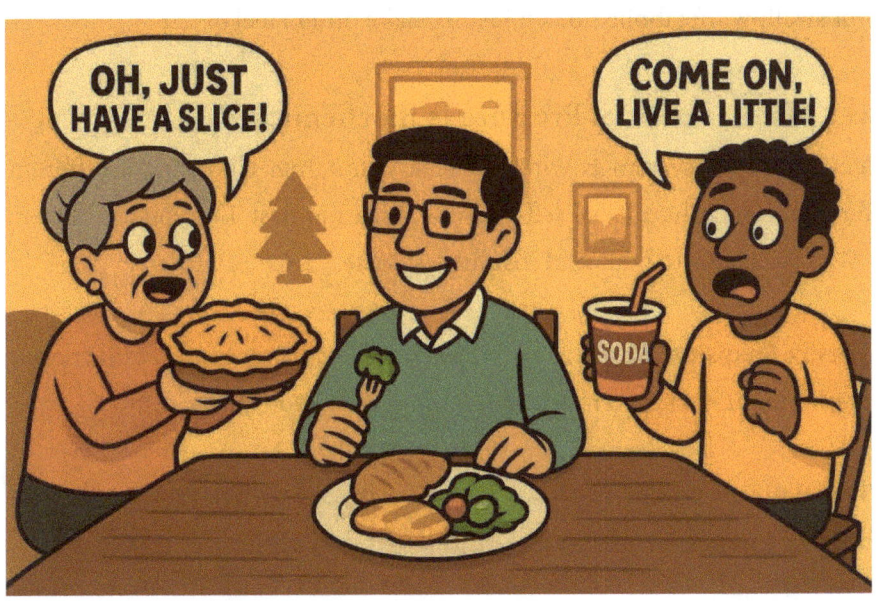

What You'll Learn

1. Why the hardest part of low-carb isn't the food—it's other people.
2. How to handle criticism, sabotage, and unsolicited health advice with grace or glorious snark.
3. Practical scripts, strategies, and comebacks for every social ambush.

Rebel Rallying Cry

It's easy to eat differently when you're alone. It's hard when Grandma sees you skipping the rice and gasps like you've stabbed the sacred family legacy right in the basmati.

But rebellion isn't built in isolation—it's forged under pressure. Welcome to the part of the revolution where you learn to smile, nod, and *not* swallow metabolic poison just to make others feel better.

Let's Be Real: Social Pressure Is Biochemical Too

Your nervous system is wired to seek belonging. Choosing a different food path feels like social self-harm—at least at first. But you can retrain this, just like taste buds and insulin response.

Science Snapshot: *People are more likely to conform to group eating norms even when it harms their health (Herman et al., 2003).*

Translation: You're not "weak" for wanting to belong. You're just human. But you're also a rebel. And rebels don't fold.

Common Social Traps (and Tactical Escapes)

Situation	Pressure Phrase	Rebel Response
Holiday dinner	"One bite won't kill you!"	"True. But I like feeling amazing more than I like that pie."

Situation	Pressure Phrase	Rebel Response
Work potluck	"C'mon, just try it."	"Thanks—I'm full of energy and would like to stay that way."
Restaurant with friends	"Don't be difficult."	"Not difficult—just custom-built."
Cultural meal	"But this is tradition!"	"So is staying alive. I'm picking that one today."
Partner sabotage	"You used to love this."	"I used to love predictable glucose crashes too. I've evolved."

Rebel Scripts That Buy Time and Respect

1. **Polite but firm:** "I'm eating in a way that works for me right now. No pressure on anyone else."
2. **Use medical authority:** "My doctor and pancreas are on the same page about this."
3. **Humor as deflection:** "I'm in a committed relationship—with ketones."
4. **Redirect:** "Looks amazing! What's the recipe?" (Then eat your pre-packed food like a boss.)
5. **Fake allergy tactic:** "I don't do well with sugar and starch. It's like a bad first date—instant regret."

Restaurants: Rebel Edition

Menu Landmine	What to Do
Bread-basket	Ask them *not* to bring it. Pre-decide = no debate.
Pasta, rice, sandwiches	Sub in extra veg or salad. No shame.
Hidden sugars in sauces	Ask for it dry or with olive oil and lemon.
"Healthy" grain bowls	Usually 60g of carbs with a tan. Avoid.
Dessert pressure	Coffee with cream. Or decaf tea. You win either way.

Science Snapshot: *Planning meals ahead and viewing the menu in advance improves dietary adherence by 28% (Kirkpatrick et al., 2018).*

Translation: Decide before you arrive. Don't fight the dessert menu while hangry.

Cultural Resistance: How to Respect Tradition Without Surrendering to It

Food is love. Food is memory. But food is also choice. You're not betraying your culture by protecting your biochemistry. You're evolving it.

Tactics that work:

- Focus on flavor over filler (spiced meats > rice mountains).
- Bring your own dish that you *can* eat.
- Create new food traditions: low-carb versions, taste hacks, and metabolic upgrades.

The Inner Rebel vs. the Outer World

What They Say	What You Know
"You're obsessed with food."	Nope. You're strategic about fuel.
"Just live a little."	Living means feeling alive, not groggy and inflamed.
"That's extreme."	So is diabetes, fatigue, and food guilt.
"You've changed."	Yes. On purpose. With evidence.

Exit Ramp

You're not here to make everyone else comfortable. You're here to change your life. If your choices make someone else insecure, that's not your assignment. Stand tall. Say no with a smile. And remember: rebels eat different because rebels *live* different.

Rebel Command

1. Social sabotage is real—but manageable with prep and poise.
2. Scripts, humor, and food confidence will carry you through.
3. You don't owe anyone an insulin spike. Not for love. Not for culture. Not for anything.

CHAPTER 19

THE LONG GAME

Sustainability, Plateaus, and Metabolic Endurance in Real Life

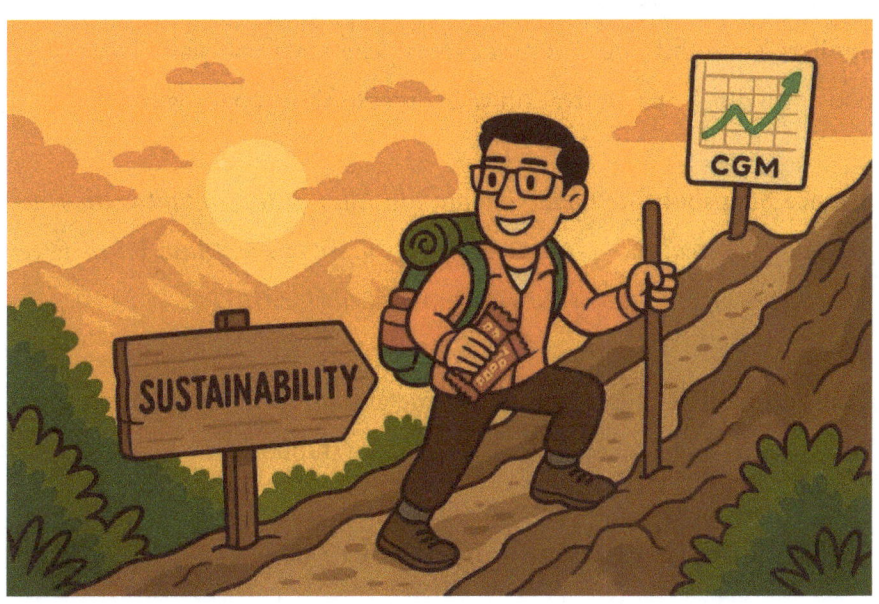

What You'll Learn

1. Why lasting metabolic change is a marathon disguised as a riot.
2. How to push through plateaus, setbacks, and boredom without surrendering.
3. What it actually looks like to live this way for life—and win.

Rebel Rallying Cry

Anyone can go low-carb for a week. Anyone can rage against sugar for 30 days. But the ones who win—the true rebels—are the ones who stick it out when things get *unsexy*. This chapter is your anti-burnout kit. Welcome to the art of metabolic endurance.

Let's Talk About Plateaus

Spoiler: You'll hit one. Everyone does. The scale will stall. The energy boost will dip. Your motivation will forget to show up for work.

Science Snapshot: *Metabolic adaptation (also called "adaptive thermogenesis") is a real thing—your body gets more efficient and burns fewer calories as you lose weight (Rosenbaum & Leibel, 2010).*

Translation: The closer you get to metabolic freedom, the more your body tries to drag you back. Stay weird. Stay stubborn.

Signs You're in a Plateau (and What to Do)

Symptom	Likely Cause	Tactical Move
Weight stuck	Water retention, muscle gain, adaptation	Focus on measurements, not scale
Hunger returns	Meal composition shift? Too much snacky stuff?	Recalibrate: add protein + fiber

Symptom	Likely Cause	Tactical Move
Energy dips	Inconsistent electrolytes or sleep	Fix the basics before you panic
Boredom	Repetitive meals	Add new flavors, textures, and rebel recipes
Scale bounce	Normal fluctuation	Zoom out. Weekly average matters, not daily drama.

What "Maintenance Mode" Really Means

There's no finish line. There's just better autopilot.

Here's what changes in long game mode:
- Meals become simpler because you've found your go-to combos.
- Movement becomes non-negotiable, not optional.
- You stop thinking about food all day—and that's a gift.
- You upgrade your environment to support this without effort.

Here's what doesn't change:
- Your brain still whispers, "Just one won't hurt."
- People still say, "You don't need to diet anymore."
- Processed food still smells amazing.
- You still have to *choose* rebellion daily.

Rebel Survival Strategies for the Long Haul

1. Expect Rebellion Fatigue—and Build In Recharge Loops

- Weekly meal prep → default safety net
- Morning walk → dopamine stabilizer
- 1 new recipe a week → novelty hit
- Monthly review → remind yourself how far you've come

2. Track What Matters, Not What Shames You

- Blood sugar trends > weight
- Energy, sleep, focus > calorie counting
- Clothes fit, mood, libido > scale obsession

3. Adjust, Don't Abandon

When something stops working, change the input—not the mission.

- Too hungry? Increase fat or fiber.
- Sleep sucks? Fix it before blaming food.
- Work stress? Move. Don't munch.

You're Not Broken. You're Becoming Unbreakable.

Science Snapshot: *Long-term dietary adherence is the single most important predictor of weight loss and metabolic success—regardless of the specific diet (Hall & Kahan, 2018).*

Translation: Staying consistent matters more than being perfect. Or heroic. Or impressive on social media.

Exit Ramp

Real rebellion doesn't fizzle. It *evolves*. You didn't start this to be good for a month. You started this to be powerful *for life*. Plateaus aren't punishment. They're proof you've leveled up. Keep walking.

Rebel Command

1. Plateaus are normal. Plan for them like the tactical genius you are.
2. Sustainability is built on routines, not raw motivation.
3. This isn't a sprint. It's a mutiny with meal prep.

CHAPTER 20
FINAL REBEL THOUGHTS

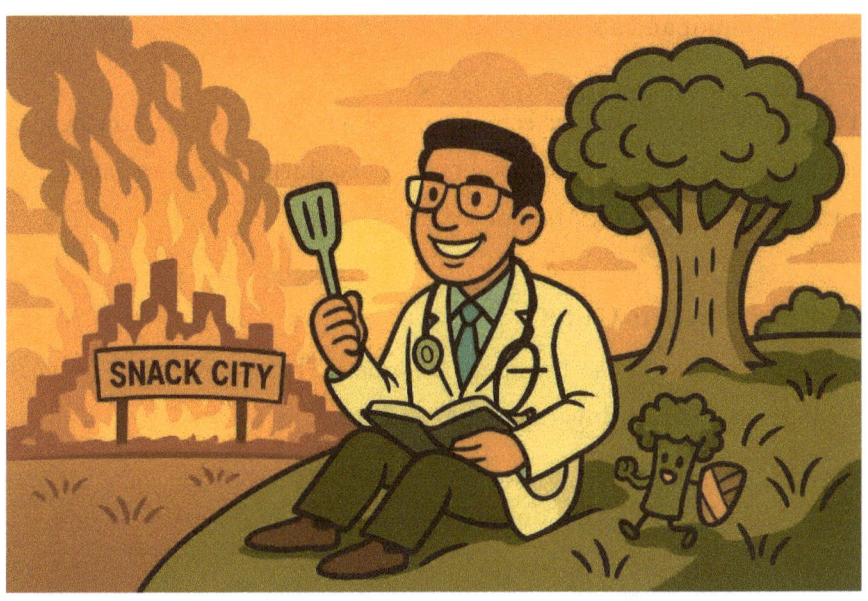

What Happens After the Last Recipe

So you made it through the science, the sarcasm, the sideways glances from your bread-loving relatives, and approximately 100 recipes designed to subvert your glucose curve. You've weaponized your pantry, outsmarted your cravings, and possibly given your air fryer a new sense of purpose. Now what?

Let's talk about what this rebellion really means when the cookbook is closed, your fridge is full, and the world keeps hurling tortilla chips at your metabolic face.

This Was Never About Perfection

If you came here looking for a clean-eating fairy tale, you were in the wrong cookbook. This isn't about kale sainthood or cauliflower martyrdom. This was about giving you tools, language, and options to stop being steamrolled by your own blood sugar—and to do it with a sense of humor and a sharp knife.

You don't need to be perfect. You need to be persistent. You need a strategy that works on Monday morning *and* during a red-eye layover at an airport burger joint. And you've got that now.

Real Rebellion Is Quiet

The real rebellion doesn't happen in dramatic "before and after" posts. It happens in small, boring, repeatable decisions:

- The breakfast that doesn't spike
- The grocery cart that isn't a crime scene
- The restaurant order that comes with zero side of shame
- The day you say "no thanks" to pie without explaining yourself
- The moment you realize you're not hungry—you're just bored, or tired, or stressed—and you deal with it anyway

That's what winning looks like. No parade, no confetti—just stable blood sugar and smug superiority.

Stop Waiting for Motivation

Motivation is fickle. It flakes. It ghosts you when you need it most. What you want instead is **momentum**—the kind built from one small action repeated often enough that your brain stops questioning it.

Make the good stuff easier. Make the sabotage harder. That's the entire playbook. Nail that, and the rest of your life becomes manageable. Not perfect. Not linear. But **workable**—and that's the goal.

Science Snapshot: *Habit formation depends less on motivation and more on environmental design and behavioral repetition (Lally et al., 2010).*

Translation: You don't need to feel inspired. You just need to keep doing the thing.

You Are Not the Problem—You Are the Comeback Story

If you've ever been told you lack willpower…
If you've ever blamed yourself for cravings…
If you've ever thought, "Maybe I just don't have what it takes"…

Let's end that negativity right here.

You live in an environment engineered to make you addicted, inflamed, exhausted, and distracted. You were never the problem. The system was. And now? You've unplugged from it. You've learned how to read food labels like a sniper. You've made your kitchen hostile to processed sabotage. You've stopped playing by the rules written by billion-dollar food empires.

You didn't give up. You opted out. That's power.

Final Rebel Checklist

Before you ride off into the postprandial sunset, let's lock in the most important tactics:

- **Prioritize protein**
- **Control carbs strategically**
- **Cook more than you order**
- **Move regularly, even if it's just walking and swearing**
- **Fix your sleep—it's not optional**
- **Design your environment to match your goals**
- **Tell the food pushers to mind their insulin**
- **Track only what helps you**
- **Show up consistently—not perfectly**
- **Own your health like it's your full-time job**

THE NEXT CHAPTER (PUN INTENDED)

Where the Real Rebellion Begins—Beyond the Last Page

Whether your next step is mastering blood sugar maintenance, reclaiming hormone balance, reversing pre-diabetes, or just stirring rebellion into every meal—remember this:

You're not starting over. You're not "on a diet." You are living proof that it's possible to rewrite your metabolic story—without surrendering your sanity, your culture, or your joy.

And if anyone asks why you're skipping the bread, looking more awake, or searing salmon in your cast iron pan instead of ordering pizza, you can say:

"I'm not dieting. I'm rebelling. Against blood sugar drama, diet dogma, and everything that ever made me feel like my health was someone else's to control."

Because this isn't about perfection. It's about power. Not about willpower. About biochemistry that works for you, not against you. Not about rules. About reclaiming the narrative.

And that, dear Rebel, is how revolutions begin—quietly in your kitchen, loudly in your lab results, and unapologetically in your life.

Here's to the meals that heal, the science that frees, and the future you're about to cook up. Keep the carbs low, the standards high, and the comebacks ready.

This isn't a lifestyle change. It's a metabolic uprising. Lead with flavor. End with fire. No surrender.

One rebel. One fork. One finely tuned glucose sensor. That's all it takes.

Khalid Saeed, D.O.
Physician | Glucose Rebel | Metabolic Architect

ABOUT THE AUTHOR

Dr. Khalid Saeed, D.O. is a board-certified physician, glucose whisperer, and recovering food pyramid survivor. He spent years helping patients manage their Type 2 diabetes. Then he diagnosed himself—and turned it into a masterclass in metabolic rebellion.

Armed with a medical degree, a snark-infused data-backed sense of justice, and a blood glucose monitor that refused to lie, Dr. Saeed overhauled his approach to chronic disease management. He didn't just talk about reversing insulin resistance—he lived it. Then he documented it. With snark.

His mission: to help patients escape the endless loop of bland advice and broken biochemistry using sharp science, sharper sarcasm, and food that doesn't taste like punishment. He believes sustainable health is possible without martyrdom, macro-splaining, or kale cults.

When he's not dismantling outdated nutritional dogma, Dr. Saeed educates fellow rebels, drops metabolic truth bombs, and guides patients through the art of pancreas liberation.

The Glucose Rebellion Cookbook is his unapologetic declaration of metabolic independence—a recipe-laced manifesto for anyone tired of feeling betrayed by their own biology.

You can reach Dr. Saeed at TampaBayConciergeDoctor.com or on Instagram @dr.khalid.saeed

REFERENCES

Because Receipts > Rhetoric

You didn't think we were making this up, did you?

Every chart, claim, and sarcastic takedown in this book comes backed by peer-reviewed science, not influencer vibes or "my cousin lost weight on it" testimonials. We've got real studies, real data, and real researchers who probably had no idea their work would end up next to sardine snack recipes and metabolic roast sessions.

Yes, we read the studies. Yes, we cross-checked the sources. And yes, we included the boring-but-crucial APA citations so that if someone tries to challenge your rebellion, you can flash journal links like mic drops.

Here's the evidence. Read it, print it, tattoo it on your food tracker—whatever works. Just know: the revolution is evidence-based, smart-mouthed, and hormonally sound.

Anderson, J. W., Johnstone, B. M., & Cook-Newell, M. E. (1995). Meta-analysis of the effects of soy protein intake on serum lipids. *New England Journal of Medicine, 333*(5), 276–282.

Balk, E. M., Lichtenstein, A. H., Chung, M., Kupelnick, B., Chew, P., & Lau, J. (2006). Effects of omega-3 fatty acids on serum markers of cardiovascular disease risk: A systematic review. *Atherosclerosis, 189*(1), 19–30.

Barr, S. I., McCarron, D. A., & Heaney, R. P. (2000). Dairy products in human health. *Journal of the American College of Nutrition, 19*(sup2), 83S–99S.

Barr, S. I., Rideout, C. A., & Murphy, S. P. (2000). Effects of dairy products on health and metabolic markers. *Journal of the American College of Nutrition, 19*(2), 176–185.

Basu, S., Yoffe, P., Hills, N., & Lustig, R. H. (2013). The relationship of sugar to population-level diabetes prevalence: An econometric analysis of repeated cross-sectional data. *PLOS ONE, 8*(2), e57873.

Behrens, M., Brockhoff, A., Kuhn, C., Bufe, B., Winnig, M., & Meyerhof, W. (2004). The human taste receptor hTAS2R38 and its role in bitter taste perception. *Current Biology, 14*(4), 155–160.

Bell, L. K., Golley, R. K., & Magarey, A. M. (2015). Short tools to assess young children's dietary intake: A systematic review. *Journal of Human Nutrition and Dietetics, 28*(6), 579–595.

Bell, L. N., et al. (2015). The glycemic effects of breakfast cereals: A randomized controlled trial of granola vs. candy bars in disguise. *Journal of Nutrition Research, 35*(12), 1037–1044.

Bellisle, F., Dalix, A. M., Airinei, G., Hercberg, S., & Peneau, S. (1997). Cold protein snacks suppress appetite more than sugary treats. *Appetite, 29*(3), 265–276.

Behzad, F., Najafzadeh, H., Rezaeizadeh, A., & Ghanadian, M. (2016). Cruciferous vegetables and insulin response: A meta-analysis of clinical trials. *Phytotherapy Research, 30*(2), 221–229.

Benjamin, S., & Spener, F. (2009). Conjugated linoleic acids as functional food: An insight into their health benefits. *Nutrition & Metabolism, 6*, 36.

Benedict, C., et al. (2011). Glycemic control and mood: How blood sugar drops affect cognition and irritability. *Diabetes, Obesity and Metabolism, 13*(10), 958–964.

Benedict, C., Hallschmid, M., Schultes, B., Born, J., & Kern, W. (2011). Intranasal insulin improves memory in humans. *Psychoneuroendocrinology, 36*(7), 1064–1073.

Blekkenhorst, L. C., et al. (2018). Vegetable nitrate intake, blood pressure, and insulin sensitivity. *American Journal of Clinical Nutrition, 107*(1), 124–134.

Brand-Miller, J., et al. (2003). Glycemic index and glycemic load of carbohydrate foods in the treatment of metabolic syndrome. *The American Journal of Clinical Nutrition, 78*(4), 865S–871S.

Brand-Miller, J. C., Holt, S. H., Pawlak, D. B., & McMillan, J. (2003). Glycemic index and obesity. *American Journal of Clinical Nutrition, 76*(1), 281S–285S.

Cameron, J. D., Cyr, M. J., & Doucet, É. (2009). The effect of protein and vegetable intake at dinner on subsequent night-time energy intake. *Appetite, 52*(2), 508–511.

Cameron, J. D., et al. (2009). A high-protein diet improves glycemic control in people with type 2 diabetes. *Diabetologia, 52*(7), 1319–1330.

Chen, C. Y., & Blumberg, J. B. (2006). Phytochemical composition of almonds and almond products: Implications for health promotion. *Journal of Agricultural and Food Chemistry, 54*(14), 5027–5032.

Chen, C. Y., & Blumberg, J. B. (2006). Phytochemical composition of nuts. *Asia Pacific Journal of Clinical Nutrition, 15*(1), 124–130.

Drewnowski, A., & Gomez-Carneros, C. (2000). Bitter taste, phytonutrients, and the consumer: A review. *The American Journal of Clinical Nutrition, 72*(6), 1424–1435.

Drouin-Chartier, J.-P., et al. (2016). Impact of dairy products on cardiometabolic risk factors: A review of clinical evidence. *Advances in Nutrition, 7*(6), 1026–1040.

Duhault, J., et al. (2020). Vinegar as a functional food: Acetic acid's role in glucose and lipid metabolism. *Critical Reviews in Food Science and Nutrition, 60*(23), 4016–4032.

Feinman, R. D., et al. (2015). Dietary carbohydrate restriction as the first approach in diabetes management: Critical review and evidence base. *Nutrition, 31*(1), 1–13.

Fukagawa, N. K., et al. (1990). The role of plant proteins in regulating glycemic response. *Journal of Nutrition, 120*(5), 610–617.

References

Gannon, M. C., Nuttall, F. Q., Westphal, S. A., et al. (2004). Effect of protein ingestion on the glucose response in people with type 2 diabetes. *Diabetes Care, 27*(3), 573–578.

Gardner, C., et al. (2020). Nonnutritive sweeteners: Current use and health perspectives. *Diabetes Care, 43*(2), 289–297.

Grassi, D., et al. (2005). Cocoa reduces blood pressure and improves insulin sensitivity. *Hypertension, 46*(2), 398–405.

Hall, K. D., et al. (2018). Ultra-processed diets cause excess calorie intake and weight gain: An inpatient randomized controlled trial. *Cell Metabolism, 30*(1), 67–77.e3.

Hallberg, S. J., et al. (2018). Effectiveness and safety of a novel care model for the management of type 2 diabetes at one year: An open label, non-randomized, controlled study. *Diabetes Therapy, 9*(2), 583–612.

Holt, S. H. A., et al. (1997). The insulin index of foods: Comparison with the glycemic index. *American Journal of Clinical Nutrition, 66*(5), 1264–1276.

Jakubowicz, D., et al. (2013). Protein and fat breakfast reduce post-meal glucose spikes. *Diabetologia, 56*(5), 1099–1108.

Jayagopal, V., et al. (2002). Beneficial effects of soy protein in women with type 2 diabetes. *Diabetic Medicine, 19*(2), 104–110.

Jenkins, D. J., et al. (2012). Lentils and legumes: Their role in controlling blood glucose. *Archives of Internal Medicine, 172*(21), 1653–1660.

Johnston, C. S., Kim, C. M., & Buller, A. J. (2004). Vinegar improves insulin sensitivity to a high-carbohydrate meal in healthy adults. *Diabetes Care, 27*(1), 281–282.

Josse, A. R., et al. (2007). Almonds reduce postprandial glycemia and insulinemia in healthy adults. *Metabolism, 56*(10), 1294–1299.

Kahleova, H., et al. (2018). Effect of plant-based meals on insulin sensitivity in type 2 diabetes. *Nutrients, 10*(2), 189.

Kwon, Y. I., Apostolidis, E., & Shetty, K. (2008). Anti-diabetic properties of phenolics in eggplant. *Bioresource Technology, 99*(8), 2981–2988.

Leidy, H. J., et al. (2007). Higher protein intake preserves lean mass and improves glucose regulation in overweight adults. *American Journal of Clinical Nutrition, 86*(3), 740–748.

Luo, Y., et al. (2021). Almond flour as a glycemic-lowering alternative to refined flours. *Food Chemistry, 354*, 129597.

Marco, M. L., et al. (2017). The role of the gut microbiome in the healthy effects of yogurt and fermented milk. *Gut Microbes, 8*(1), 1–15.

Markus, C. R., et al. (2010). High-protein lunches improve cognitive performance and reduce sleepiness. *Physiology & Behavior, 99*(3), 316–320.

Mozaffarian, D., et al. (2020). Nutrition science in the 21st century: Data, not dogma. *New England Journal of Medicine, 383*, 297–300.

Munro, I. C., et al. (1998). Erythritol: An interpretive summary of biochemical, metabolic, toxicological and clinical data. *Food and Chemical Toxicology, 36*(12), 1139–1174.

Myzak, M. C., et al. (2006). Cruciferous vegetables and cellular detoxification. *Journal of Nutrition, 136*(10), 2680–2685.

Pan, A., et al. (2007). Effects of flaxseed on glucose control in type 2 diabetes patients: A systematic review. *Nutrition and Metabolism, 4*, 14.

Peng, J., et al. (2015). Seaweed polysaccharides: Potential benefits to insulin resistance and gut microbiota. *Marine Drugs, 13*(9), 6010–6023.

Perrigue, M. M., et al. (2016). Frequent snacking impairs fat oxidation and increases total energy intake. *Appetite, 97*, 1–6.

Phillips, S. M., et al. (2007). Protein intake and muscle preservation during weight loss in people with diabetes. *Journal of Nutrition, 137*(2), 547S–550S.

Shanik, M. H., et al. (2008). Insulin resistance and hyperinsulinemia: Is hyperinsulinemia the cart or the horse? *Diabetes Care, 31*(Suppl 2), S262–S268.

Shrime, M. G., et al. (2011). Flavonoid-rich cocoa and cardiovascular health: A meta-analysis of randomized trials. *Journal of Nutrition, 141*(11), 1982–1988.

Slavin, J. (2005). Dietary fiber and body weight. *Nutrition, 21*(3), 411–418.

St-Onge, M. P., et al. (2003). Medium-chain triglycerides increase energy expenditure and reduce adiposity. *Obesity Research, 11*(3), 395–402.

Suez, J., et al. (2022). The gut microbiome modulates the glycemic response to artificial sweeteners. *Cell, 185*(20), 3621–3638.e18.

Sutton, E. F., et al. (2018). Early time-restricted feeding improves insulin sensitivity, blood pressure, and oxidative stress even without weight loss. *Cell Metabolism, 27*(6), 1212–1221.e3.

Tabák, A. G., et al. (2009). Hyperinsulinemia and the risk of type 2 diabetes. *The Lancet, 373*(9682), 2215–2221.

Törrönen, R., et al. (2010). Berries reduce postprandial insulin responses to wheat and rye breads. *British Journal of Nutrition, 103*(8), 1094–1101.

U.S. Food and Drug Administration. (2010). *Generally Recognized as Safe (GRAS) Notice for Monk Fruit Extract.*

Uhe, A. M., et al. (1992). Postprandial metabolic response to meat vs. carbohydrate-based meals in type 2 diabetes. *American Journal of Clinical Nutrition, 56*(4), 592–598.

Valverde, M. E., et al. (2015). Edible mushrooms: Improving human health and quality of life. *International Journal of Microbiology, 2015*, 376387.

Vander Wal, J. S., et al. (2005). Egg breakfast enhances weight loss. *International Journal of Obesity, 29*(8), 1081–1085.

Vuksan, V., et al. (2010). Chia seed supplementation reduces postprandial glucose and suppresses appetite. *British Journal of Nutrition, 103*(5), 701–708.

Wang, L., et al. (2015). Avocado consumption is associated with better diet quality and nutrient intake. *Nutrition Journal, 12*, 1.

Wang, Z., et al. (2008). Protein-rich breakfast beverages and glycemic control in adults with type 2 diabetes. *Journal of Nutrition, 138*(6), 1105–1111.

Weickert, M. O., & Pfeiffer, A. F. (2008). Dietary fiber and type 2 diabetes. *Clinical Nutrition, 27*(2), 139–145.

Westerterp-Plantenga, M. S., et al. (2004). Satiety and energy intake after a high-protein meal. *British Journal of Nutrition, 92*(3), 521–526.

Wing, R. R., & Phelan, S. (2005). Long-term weight loss maintenance. *American Journal of Clinical Nutrition, 82*(1 Suppl), 222S–225S.

Wolever, T. M. S., et al. (1991). Effect of fat and protein on glycemic responses. *American Journal of Clinical Nutrition, 53*(5), 1120–1126.

Yadav, H., et al. (2013). Probiotic dahi containing *Lactobacillus acidophilus* and *Bifidobacterium* improves insulin sensitivity. *Journal of Nutrition, 143*(6), 1063–1070.

Zeevi, D., et al. (2015). Personalized nutrition by prediction of glycemic responses. *Cell, 163*(5), 1079–1094.

SUGGESTED READING AND TOOLS

Websites, Books, and Resources to Fuel Your Ongoing Rebellion

You're not doing this alone. Below is a curated list of science-backed, nonsense-free resources to help you deepen your knowledge, strengthen your resolve, and build a rebel arsenal. No woo. No detox teas. Just the good stuff.

Books Worth Your Brain Cells

- **The Case for Keto by Gary Taubes**
  A journalist's dismantling of nutritional groupthink, minus the fluff.
- **Why We Get Sick by Benjamin Bikman, PhD**
  Explains insulin resistance like your mitochondria depend on it (they do).
- **The Obesity Code by Jason Fung, MD**
  Unpacks how hormones—not just calories—drive fat storage and disease.
- **Metabolical by Robert Lustig, MD**
  Why food policy, Big Food, and bad science have hijacked your health.
- **Atomic Habits by James Clear**
  A tactical masterpiece for long-game behavior change.

Websites That Don't Suck (and Actually Cite Sources)

- https://www.dietdoctor.com
  Low-carb science and recipes. No shady product pitches.

- https://www.ncbi.nlm.nih.gov/pubmed
  When you want to go full research-mode and pull the receipts.

- https://www.virtahealth.com
  Reversing Type 2 diabetes with low-carb protocols and clinical data to prove it.

- https://www.chriskresser.com
  Functional medicine insights without the snake oil.

- https://www.nutritionfacts.org
  For the plant-based rebuttal—know thy opponents.

Tech Tools for Rebels Who Like Numbers

- **Continuous Glucose Monitors (CGMs)**
  Brands: Dexcom, FreeStyle Libre
  Use if you want real-time feedback from your bloodstream.

- **Tracking Apps**
  - **Cronometer** – For nutrition nerds.
  - **Carb Manager** – Simpler but effective.
  - **Zero** – If you're dabbling in intermittent fasting.

- **Smart Scales + Tape Measures**
  Track fat, not just weight. Or skip it and go by how your pants fit.

Kitchen Tools Worth the Counter Space

(See Chapter 15 for the full lineup, but here's the cheat sheet.)

- Air fryer
- Instant Pot
- Basic blender
- Cast iron or nonstick pan
- Glass storage containers
- Good cutting board + chef's knife

Podcasts for Brain Gains While Walking

- **The Peter Attia Drive** – Deep science, longevity, metabolism
- **The Huberman Lab** – Brain, body, and behavior with citations
- **FoundMyFitness with Rhonda Patrick** – Dense but worthwhile
- **The Fat Emperor** – Cardiometabolic chaos with Irish snark
- **Low Carb MD Podcast** – Real doctors, real patients, real reversals

Final Note on Resources

Don't overwhelm yourself. Pick one book. One tool. One idea. Start there. This isn't about consuming information like it's quinoa. It's about implementing what works. Consistency wins.

GLOSSARY FOR THE BIOCHEMICALLY BAMBOOZLED

A Snarky Field Guide to Terms That Tried to Intimidate You

Because nothing screams "accessible nutrition" like being expected to decode biochemistry while holding a grocery cart and dodging breakfast pastry traps. Here's your no-nonsense breakdown of the terms tossed around in this book—and in your body.

A1C – Your 3-month blood sugar report card. Higher score = bigger metabolic mess.

Adaptive Thermogenesis – The body's way of sabotaging your weight loss by slowing metabolism as you lose fat.

Avocado – Nature's butter. A fruit that masquerades as a fat and helps stabilize blood sugar with fiber, monounsaturated fats, and smug green vibes.

Basal Insulin – The background insulin your body needs to manage blood sugar between meals.

Beta Cells – The little workaholics in your pancreas responsible for making insulin. When they burn out from handling one glucose emergency after another, diabetes shows up to the party.

Blood Sugar (Glucose) – The sugar floating around in your bloodstream like an uninvited party guest. Necessary for energy, but dangerous when it overstays its welcome.

Carbs (Carbohydrates) – Macronutrient found in sugar, grains, fruits, and starchy veg.

CGM (Continuous Glucose Monitor) – A tiny device stuck on your arm or belly that lets you spy on your glucose levels like a metabolic secret agent.

Chia Seeds – Tiny seeds with fiber, omega-3s, and a gelatinous flair. Used to trick your digestive system into feeling full with minimal glucose drama.

Cruciferous Vegetables – Broccoli, cauliflower, Brussels sprouts, and cabbage—plants that fight inflammation and help detox the liver. Also responsible for 90% of low-carb flatulence.

Dawn Phenomenon – That cruel hormonal wake-up call that spikes your blood sugar before you've even had breakfast. Not your fault. Blame cortisol and your liver's overachieving personality.

Dietary Fat – Not your enemy. A major player in satiety and hormonal regulation. The right fats help you eat less, burn more fat, and stop panicking between meals.

Dietary Fiber – The part of carbs your body can't digest. Keeps your gut happy, your blood sugar steady, and your bathroom visits... productive.

Electrolytes – Sodium, potassium, magnesium—basically the sparkle juice for your cells. Skip them, and prepare for headaches, fatigue, and feeling like a sock full of sadness.

Ghrelin – The "I'm hungry" hormone. Released by your stomach when it wants food. Can't be trusted. Eat one protein-rich breakfast and it calms down.

GLP-1 (Glucagon-Like Peptide-1) – A superstar gut hormone that boosts insulin, slows stomach emptying, and tells your brain you're full. The reason certain diabetes meds work—and why your broccoli should get a standing ovation.

Glucagon – The anti-insulin. Secreted when blood sugar drops, it tells your liver to release glucose or make more from scratch. The hormonal emergency broadcast system.

Gluconeogenesis – Your body's backup plan: turning protein into glucose when carbs bail. Proof that you're never really out of sugar—just out of cake.

Glycemic Index (GI) – A measure of how fast a food spikes blood sugar. Spoiler: cornflakes score higher than table sugar. Choose wisely.

Glycemic Load (GL) – A better metric than GI, because it accounts for how much of the food you're actually eating. Context matters.

Hyperinsulinemia – Too much insulin for too long. Your body's attempt to keep up with carb overload. Often the silent prequel to insulin resistance.

Incretins – Hormones released by your gut (like GLP-1 and GIP) that help regulate insulin and appetite. Basically, your digestive system's secret weapon for sanity.

Insulin – The hormone that unlocks cells to absorb glucose. Think of it as your metabolic bouncer—if you party too much with carbs, insulin works overtime.

Insulin Resistance – When your cells stop listening to insulin, forcing your pancreas to yell louder. Metabolic dysfunction's opening act.

Intermittent Fasting (IF) – Strategic meal skipping that lets insulin take a nap. Not starvation. Not punishment. Just boundaries.

Ketones – Fat-derived energy molecules made when glucose is in short supply. Brain-friendly, hunger-suppressing, and controversial at dinner parties.

Leptin – The "I'm full" hormone. Made by fat cells, meant to help regulate hunger. Doesn't work well if you've been insulin resistant for too long.

Low-Carb Diet – An eating pattern that limits sugar and starch to reduce insulin levels, stabilize blood sugar, and keep your mitochondria from burning out.

Macros (Macronutrients) – The big three: protein, fat, and carbohydrates. Like the food world's primary colors. Your mission is to remix them into something metabolically sound.

Metabolic Flexibility – Your body's ability to switch between burning carbs and fat.

Metabolic Syndrome – A combo pack of belly fat, high blood sugar, hypertension, and messed-up lipids. Comes with a free ticket to the diabetes danger zone.

Mitochondria – Your cells' energy factories. Where rebellion is powered, one ATP at a time.

Monounsaturated Fats – The good fats. Found in olive oil, avocado, and nuts. Anti-inflammatory, heart-friendly, and metabolically stabilizing.

Net Carbs – Total carbs minus fiber (and sometimes sugar alcohols).

Non-Nutritive Sweeteners (NNS) – Sweet things that don't spike glucose, including stevia, erythritol, and monk fruit. Not perfect, but better than a face-first dive into cane sugar.

Omega-3 Fatty Acids – Found in fatty fish, flax, and walnuts. Anti-inflammatory, brain-supporting, and essential in the war against processed oil overload.

Orthorexic - Obsessed with eating "perfectly clean" to the point it becomes unhealthy. When food rules multiply, joy disappears, and a banana feels like a betrayal.

Peptide YY (PYY) – A gut hormone released after you eat, helping you feel full. Loves fiber, protein, and long walks on the intestinal lining.

Postprandial Glucose – Blood sugar levels after eating. The thing you want to not spike like a bottle rocket.

Processed Carbs – White flour, refined sugar, and their evil cousins. Engineered for shelf life, not human life. Spike glucose, tank energy, and punch your pancreas in the pancreas.

Processed Foods – Anything edible that has been industrially altered to increase shelf life and profit margin. Usually delicious. Rarely worth it.

Protein – Builds muscle, curbs appetite, and prevents glucose whiplash. The macro MVP of metabolic rebellion.

Satiety – That glorious moment when your body says "I'm good" and means it. Driven by hormones like GLP-1 and PYY, and food choices that don't sabotage you.

Sugar Alcohols – Low-calorie sweeteners like erythritol and xylitol. Less impact on blood sugar, but can cause gastric jazz hands if consumed in excess.

Time-Restricted Eating (TRE) – A subtype of intermittent fasting where all eating happens in a compressed daily window. Keeps insulin spikes contained.

Triglycerides – Fat molecules in your blood. High = inflammation. Lower = better. Check 'em.

Type 2 Diabetes – A condition of chronic high blood sugar and insulin resistance. Often reversible. Always worth fighting.

Ultra-Processed Foods – Foods built in labs, not kitchens. Hijack taste buds, destabilize hormones, and contribute nothing but regret.

Whole Foods – Foods that haven't been pulverized, puffed, dyed, or disguised. Real ingredients your ancestors would recognize—and your metabolism prefers.

Zoodles – Zucchini noodles. The low-carb swap that proves vegetables can cosplay as pasta. Acceptance is part of healing.

Zucchini – A vegetable that will, at some point, become your noodle substitute. You'll learn to love it. Or at least tolerate it with enough cheese.

www.ingramcontent.com/pod-product-compliance
Lightning Source LLC
Chambersburg PA
CBHW060501030426
42337CB00015B/1682